Theranostics - An Old Concept in New Clothing

Edited by Elisabeth Eppard

Published in London, United Kingdom

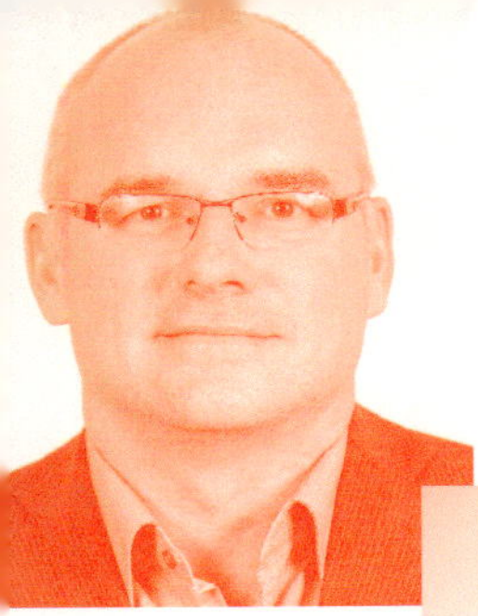
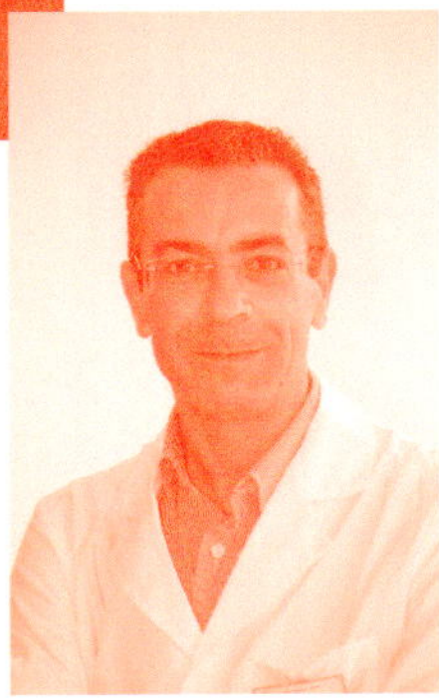
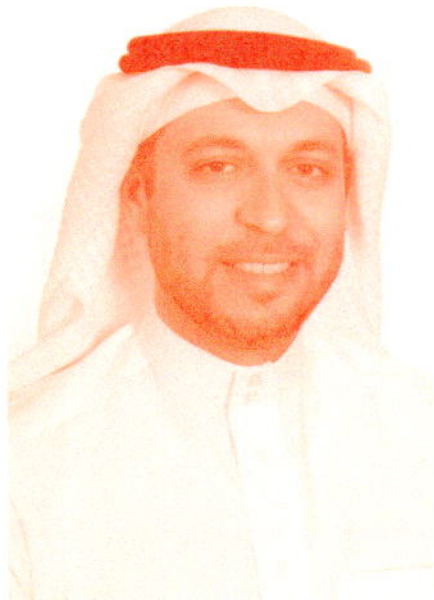
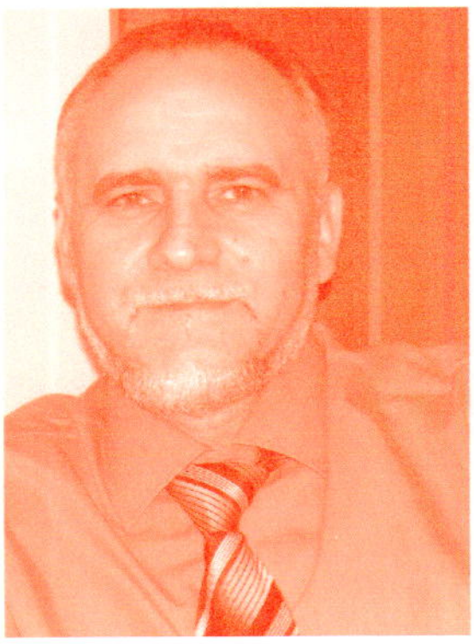
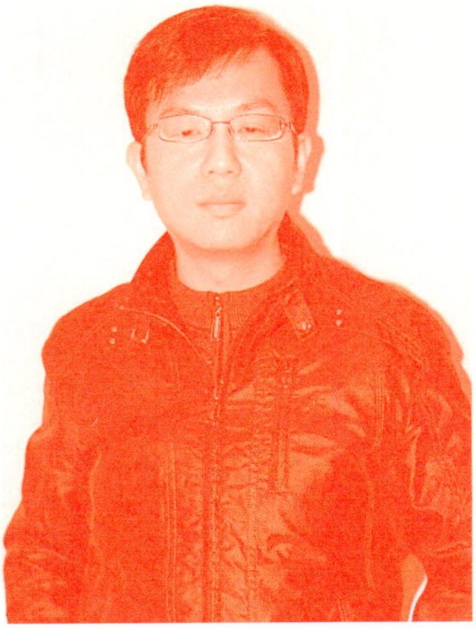
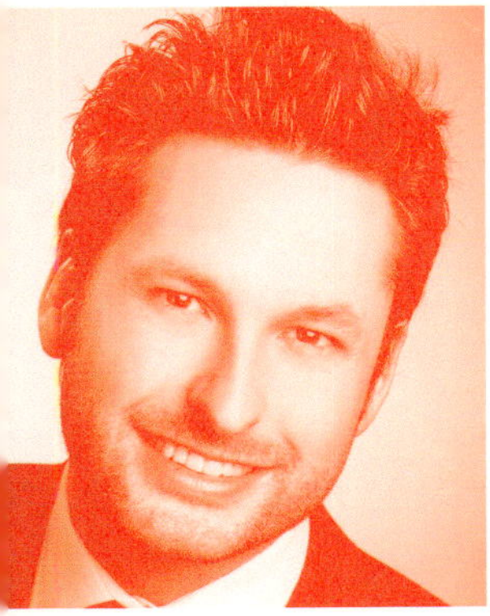
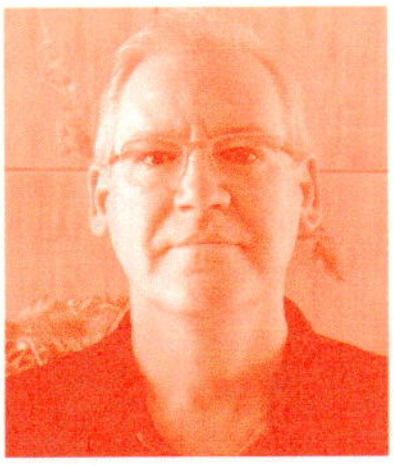

IntechOpen

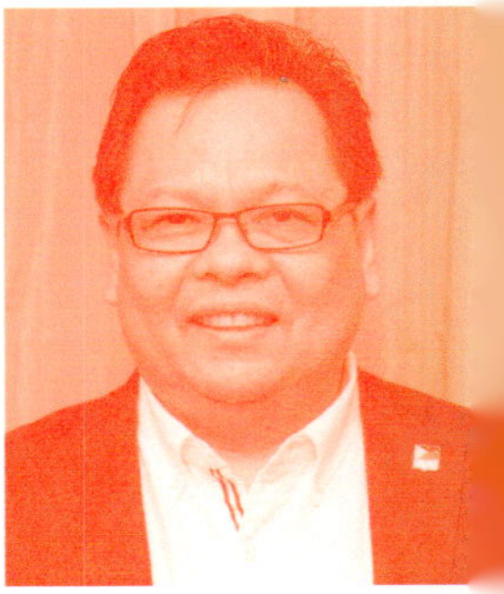
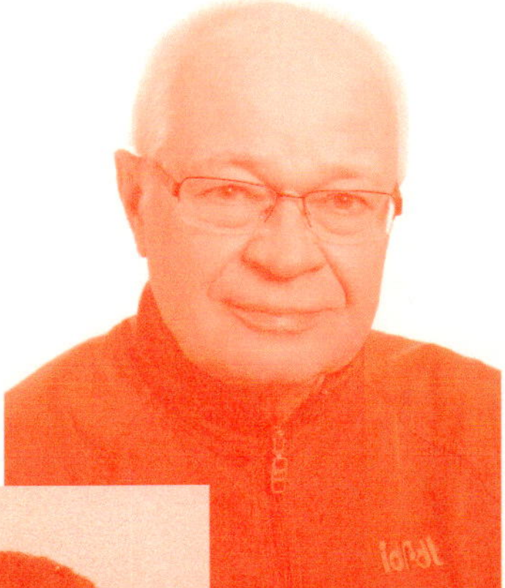
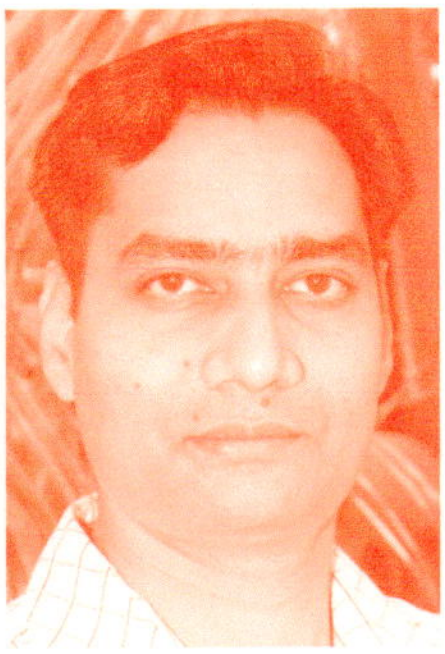
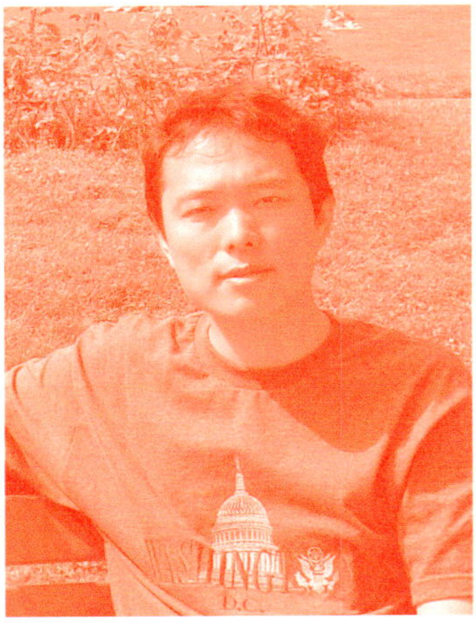
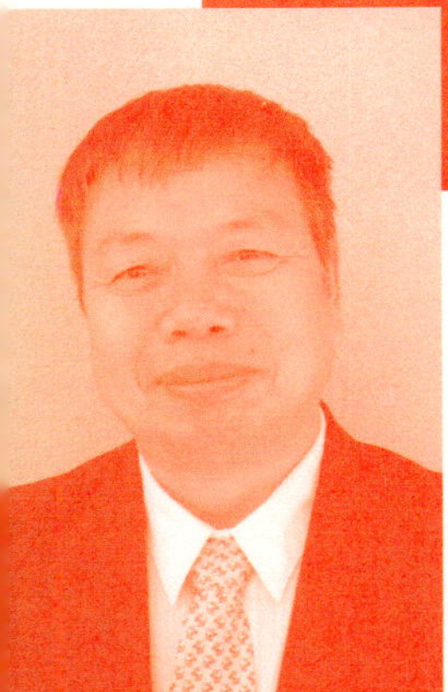
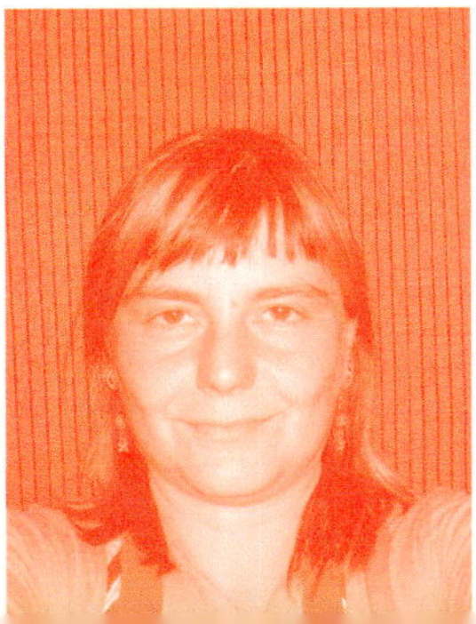

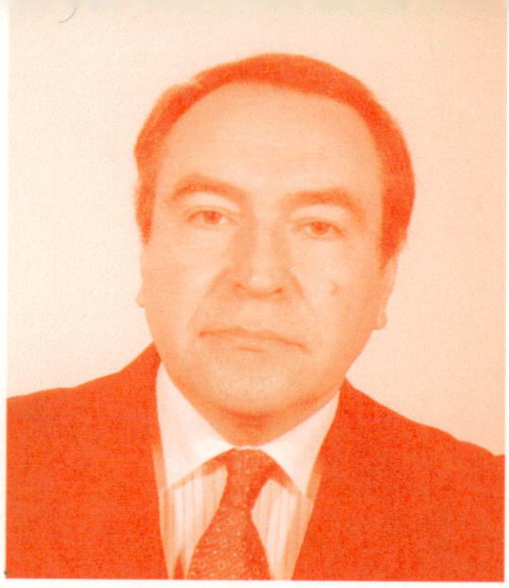
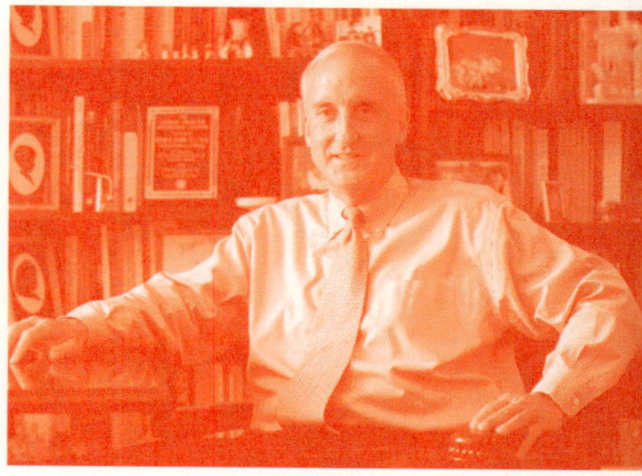
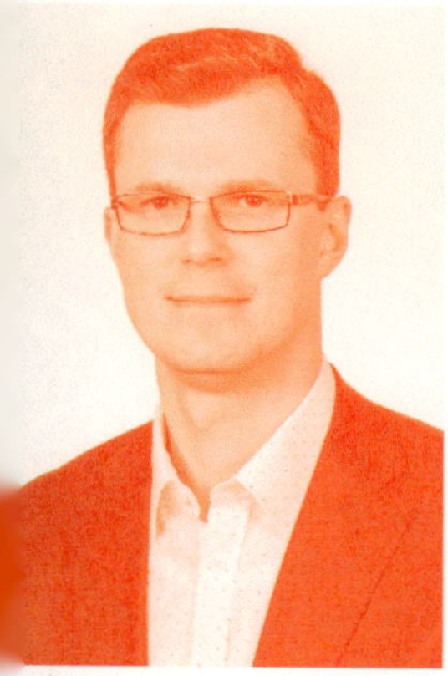
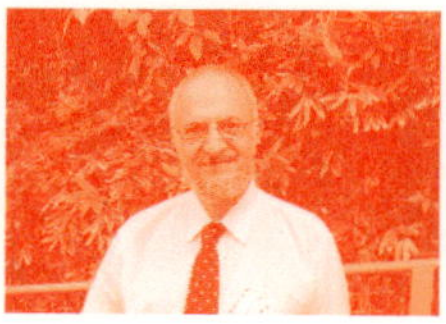
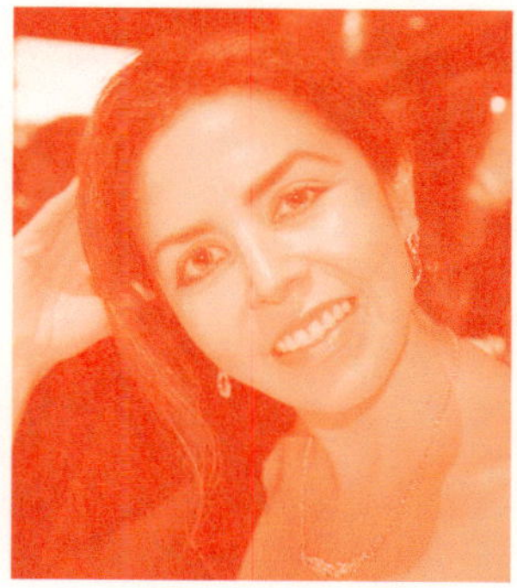

Supporting open minds since 2005

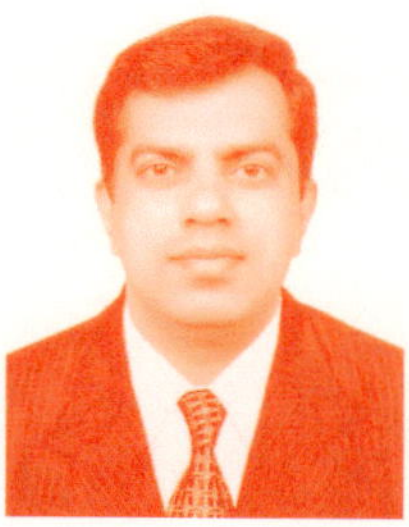
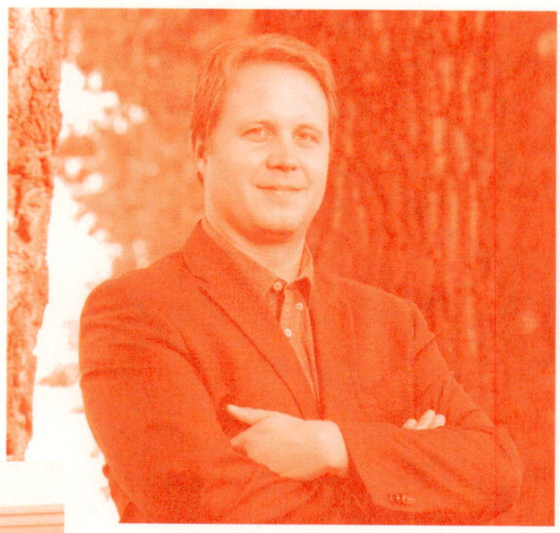
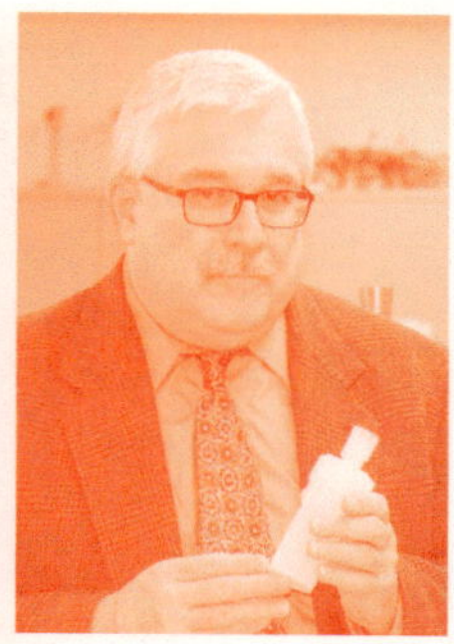
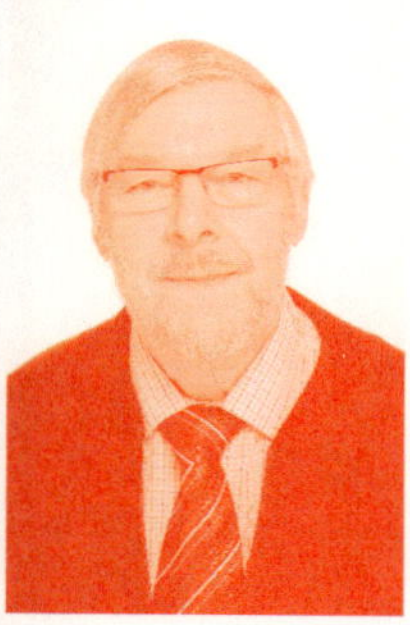
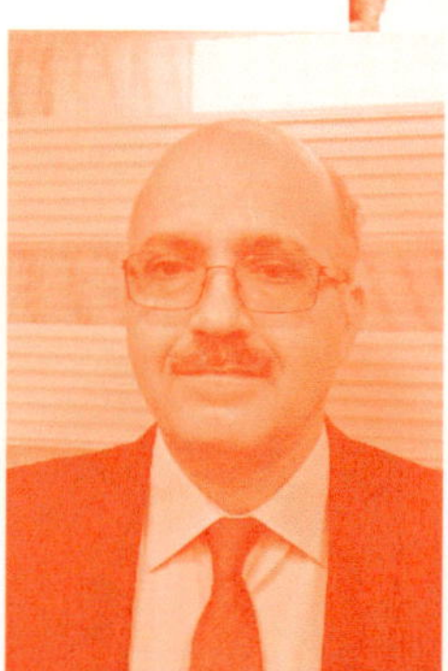
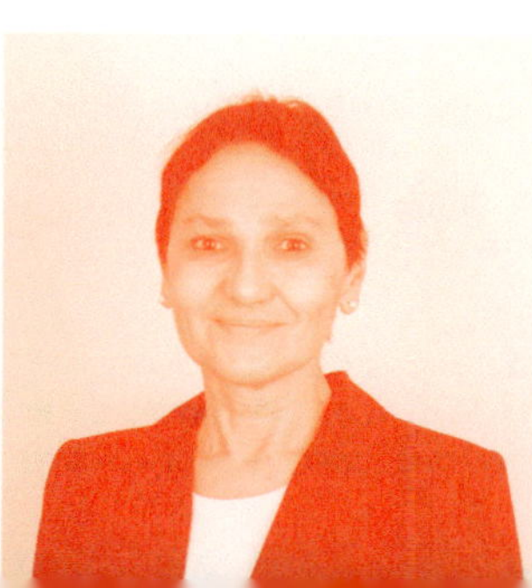
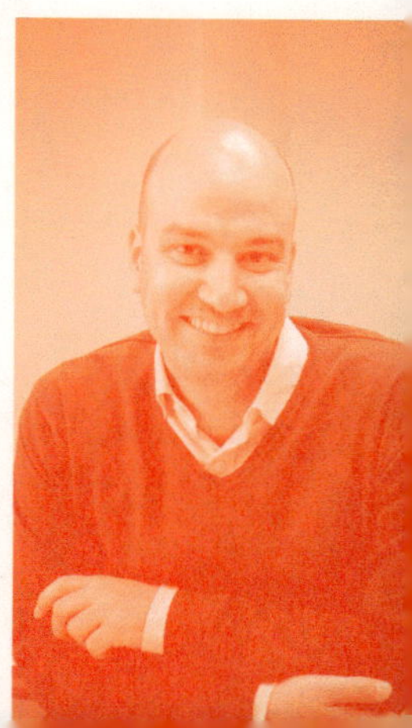

Theranostics - An Old Concept in New Clothing
http://dx.doi.org/10.5772/intechopen.91073
Edited by Elisabeth Eppard

Contributors
Arghya Sett, Renata Mikolajczak, Justyna Pijarowska-Kruszyna, Piotr Garnuszek, Clemens Decristoforo, Chunying Liu, Changqing Su, Xuejing Lin, Marlene Lúcio, Eduarda Fernandes, Hugo Gonçalves, Maria Elisabete C.D. Real Oliveira, Andreia Ferreira de Castro Gomes, Sofia Machado, Sameer Kumar, Aswini Poyyakkara, Sruthi Thekkeveedu, Sharath Shankar, Matthias M. Herth, Markus Staudt, Christian Bernard Matthijs Poulie

First published in London, United Kingdom, 2021 by IntechOpen
IntechOpen is the global imprint of INTECHOPEN LIMITED, registered in England and Wales, registration number: 11086078, 5 Princes Gate Court, London, SW7 2QJ, United Kingdom
Printed in Croatia

British Library Cataloguing-in-Publication Data
A catalogue record for this book is available from the British Library

Additional hard and PDF copies can be obtained from orders@intechopen.com

Theranostics - An Old Concept in New Clothing
Edited by Elisabeth Eppard
p. cm.
Print ISBN 978-1-83962-783-5
Online ISBN 978-1-83962-788-0
eBook (PDF) ISBN 978-1-83962-789-7

For EU product safety concerns:
IN TECH d.o.o., Prolaz Marije Krucifikse Kozulić 3, 51000 Rijeka, Croatia, info@intechopen.com or visit our website at intechopen.com.

Meet the editor

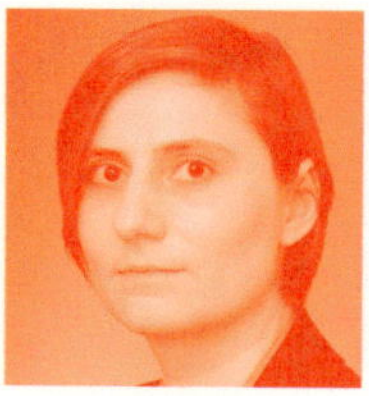

Dr. Elisabeth Eppard is a radiochemist working on the development and process implementation of new compounds for theranostic application. In 2013 she obtained her Ph.D. under Prof. Rösch at the Institute of Nuclear Chemistry, Johannes Gutenberg University Mainz, Germany, where she worked on radiometal-based radiopharmaceuticals. After four years as a junior research group leader in the Department of Nuclear Medicine, University Hospital Bonn, Germany, Dr. Eppard joined Positronpharma SA, Santiago, Chile, as a senior scientist in 2018. There she was responsible for research and clinical applications based on 68Ga-, 44Sc-, and 177Lu-labelled theranostics. Since 2021, she has been a radiochemist in the Department of Nuclear Medicine, University Hospital Magdeburg, Germany, where she is continuing her research.

Contents

Preface

In recent years the paradigm of "one-size-fits-all" in medicine has shifted successively to more patient-oriented treatment strategies [1, 2]. The aim of this personalized approach is to treat the right patient at the right time with the right drug to achieve maximum effect with minimal adverse effects. According to the definition of the U.S. National Cancer Institute, personalized medicine is "a form of medicine that uses information about a person's own genes or proteins to prevent, diagnose, or treat disease."

To meet this challenge, individual patient treatment and accurate diagnosis is indispensable. This includes, but is not limited to, characterization, staging, and quantification of the underlying disease, all of which guide physician decisions for optimal treatment planning. Beyond that, deeper knowledge and understanding of the individual properties and differences of the same disease in different patients paves the way for the development of tailored drugs and for the treatment of the individual patient's needs.

In this context, so-called theranostics has importance. Though the term was established in 2002 as a portmanteau of "therapy" and "diagnostics," the concept itself has been adopted elsewhere and explored for decades [3]. Originally describing "any material that combines the modalities of therapy and diagnostic imaging," theranostics now commonly refers to image-guided therapy [4].

Since the pioneering work of Saul Hertz (1905–1950), the father of theranostics, who first applied radioactive iodine for therapy in 1941 and influenced strongly the management paradigm for diseases of the thyroid [5], the field has evolved and expanded greatly. Growing knowledge about the genesis of a disease and more sophisticated diagnostic and therapeutic techniques promote the research and development of new theranostic materials and, ultimately, drugs.

This book presents a selection of new developments in the area of theranostics and provides a comprehensive overview of the state of the art in this exciting discipline.

Elisabeth Eppard
Klinik für Radiologie und Nuklearmedizin/
Universitätsklinikum Magdeburg A.ö.R.,
Magdeburg, Germany

References

[1] La Thangue NB, Kerr DJ. Predictive biomarkers: a paradigm shift towards personalized cancer medicine. Nat Rev Clin Oncol 2011; 8(10):587-96. Available from: URL: https://www.nature.com/articles/nrclinonc.2011.121.

[2] Diamandis M, White NMA, Yousef GM. Personalized medicine: marking a new epoch in cancer patient management. Mol Cancer Res 2010; 8(9):1175-87. Available from: URL: https://mcr.aacrjournals.org/content/8/9/1175.short.

[3] Reinventing pharma: the theranostic revolution; 2002.

[4] Luk BT, Zhang L. Current advances in polymer-based nanotheranostics for cancer treatment and diagnosis. ACS Appl. Mater. Interfaces 2014; 6(24):21859-73.

[5] Ehrhardt JD, Güleç S. Radyoaktif İyot Teranostiğinin Kısa Hikayesi: Nükleer Ontolojinin Kökenleri. Mol Imaging Radionucl Ther 2020; 29(3):88-97.

Section 1

Theranostic Radiopharmaceuticals

Chapter 1

Radiopharmaceutical Precursors for Theranostics

Justyna Pijarowska-Kruszyna, Piotr Garnuszek, Clemens Decristoforo and Renata Mikołajczak

Abstract

Due to the complex nomenclature used in various regulations and guidance documents, the understanding of radiopharmaceutical precursor's definition might be challenging. Depending on the context it could be interpreted as the substance which becomes a radiopharmaceutical after radiolabeling with a radionuclide of choice or a radionuclide which is used for radiolabeling of that substance. In this Chapter we present and discuss the requirements for precursors which are used in the preparation of theranostic radiopharmaceuticals, in particular for preparation of new radiopharmaceuticals for clinical trials within the EU. In discussion on the available methods for assessing the quality of radiopharmaceutical precursors and on the specified limits the reference to Ph. Eur. is made. Since the EANM guidelines for in-house preparation of radiopharmaceuticals also specify the need for testing the quality of radiopharmaceutical precursors, information provided herein might help the radiopharmacist working on the development of new theranostic agents to adequately define identity, strength, quality, purity and stability of the final radiopharmaceutical preparation.

Keywords: radiopharmaceutical precursors, radionuclide precursor, chemical precursor, peptides, IMPD, clinical trials

1. Introduction

This chapter deals with regulatory considerations related to radiopharmaceutical precursors within Europe. Outside, different aspects may apply, with the exception of certain harmonized documents. Radiopharmaceuticals are considered a safe class of medicinal products. Due to the small chemical quantities administered they are not expected to exhibit any measurable pharmacological effect [1]. However, since they are radioactive, the rules for minimizing the risk associated with the use of ionizing radiation to the patients and to the personnel must be observed. Depending on the chemical and physical properties, radiopharmaceuticals are used in major clinical areas for diagnostics and/or therapy [2]. As defined by the European Pharmacopeia (Ph. Eur.) general monograph (0125) *radiopharmaceutical preparations or radiopharmaceuticals* are medicinal products which, when ready for use, contain one or more radionuclides (radioactive isotopes) included for a medicinal purpose [3]. Importantly, they can also have the form of kits for radio-pharmaceutical preparation, radionuclide generators and radionuclide precursors.

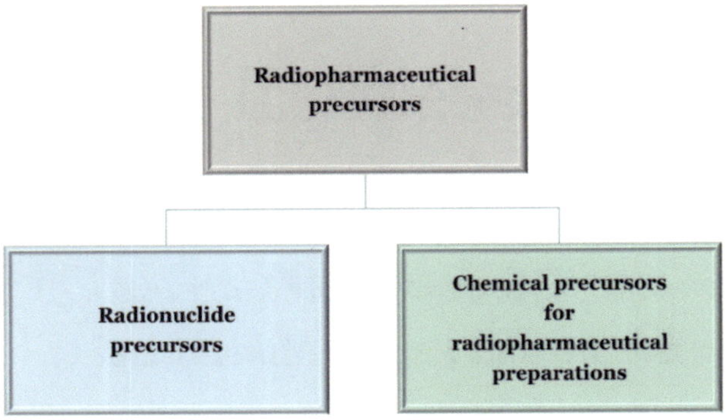

Figure 1.
Radiopharmaceutical precursors according to Ph. Eur.

For the latter it is understood that they are not used in patients as such but only after attaching them to the suitable pharmaceutical vector. Although according to Ph. Eur. monograph (0125) *radionuclide precursor* is any radionuclide produced for radiolabeling of another substance prior to administration, and according to Ph. Eur. general monograph (2902) the substance, which is used as such vector, is defined as a *chemical precursor for radiopharmaceutical preparations* [4], the term *radiopharmaceutical precursor* is used interchangeably for either of the two above defined precursors (**Figure 1**).

2. Current regulatory framework

Given the complex nomenclature used in various regulations and guidance documents, the understanding of radiopharmaceutical precursor's definition might be challenging. Depending on the context it could be interpreted as the substance which becomes a radiopharmaceutical after radiolabeling with a radionuclide of choice or a radionuclide which is used for radiolabeling of that substance. Therefore, the quality requirements and test methods specifications of precursors for use in preparation of theranostic radiopharmaceuticals can be discussed only in the light of current regulatory framework.

The preparation and use of radiopharmaceuticals are regulated by number of directives, regulations and rules. These documents may be classified with respect to the status of radiopharmaceutical preparation:

1. radiopharmaceuticals with marketing authorization (MA), regulated by:

    - Directives: 2001/83/EC [5], 2003/94/EC [6], 2004/27/EC [7];

    - GMP guidelines and annexes [8];

2. radiopharmaceuticals to be used in clinical trials (CT), regulated by:

    - Directives: 2001/20/EC [9], 2003/94/EC [6], 2005/28/EC [10]

    - and soon to be replaced by Regulation EU No 536/2014 [11];

3. unlicensed radiopharmaceuticals extemporaneously (just before use) prepared, not for CT [12, 13].

Radiopharmaceuticals with marketing authorization (MA) meet the requirements of GMP Annex 3 (Manufacture of Radiopharmaceuticals) [8] and EMA Guideline on Radiopharmaceuticals [12]. For the small scale preparation of radiopharmaceuticals outside the marketing authorization the guide of the Pharmaceutical Inspection Convention and Pharmaceutical Inspection Co-operation Scheme (PIC/S) [14], the Guidelines on Good Radiopharmacy Practice (CRPP) issued by the Radiopharmacy Committee of European Association of Nuclear Medicine (EANM) [13] and the Chapter 5.19. Extemporaneous preparation of radiopharmaceutical preparations of the Ph. Eur. [15] are setting standards for good practices.

The translation of new radiopharmaceuticals from the preclinical stage into clinical trials requires appropriate quality assessment essential to ensure efficacy and safety of both drug substance and drug product [16, 17]. The specific regulatory framework for the use of radiopharmaceuticals in clinical trials has been established in Europe [9, 11, 18]. From the radiopharmaceutical development perspective, the essential step is the preparation of an Investigational Medicinal Product Dossier (IMPD). This document includes information related to the chemical and pharmaceutical quality of the drug substance and drug product, as well as non-clinical data related to pharmacology, pharmacokinetics, radiation dosimetry and toxicology [19]. IMPD contains two main sections related to the production and quality control of the radiopharmaceutical: the drug substance (the active pharmaceutical ingredient, or API) and the drug product.

An *active pharmaceutical ingredient (API)* is defined as any substance or mixture of substances intended to be used in the manufacture of a drug product. Such substances are intended to provide pharmacological activity or other direct effect in the diagnosis as well as treatment of disease or to affect the structure and function of the body. Radiopharmaceutical preparations are often formulated using predefined radionuclide precursors and chemical precursors. If such a preparation does not need a purification step prior to its administration to the patient, both precursors used in the synthesis are considered to be an API in the drug substance part of IMPD. This in particular applies to precursors for theranostic applications where a radiometal is used to radiolabel a vector targeting the receptor, e.g. peptide. On the other hand, chemical precursors used in the manufacture of radiopharmaceuticals, which are purified after the radiolabeling process, are defined as API starting material (e.g. chemical precursors for most F-18 and C-11 PET radiopharmaceuticals).

The manufacture of APIs should be carried out following general GMP requirements. In a GMP-based system, all processes are defined, systematically reviewed, and shown to be capable of consistently providing medicinal products of the required quality and complying with their specifications [20]. Written and approved protocols specifying critical steps, acceptance criteria, must be in place. Process validation is a crucial part of GMP, meaning that all critical steps of manufacturing processes as well as significant changes to these processes are validated. It should be noted that the requirements for validations differ depending whether marketing authorization, clinical trials or in-house preparation of radiopharmaceuticals are planned (see also **Figure 2.**) [21]. The qualification and validation aspects related to the small-scale "in house" preparation of radiopharmaceuticals are covered in the EANM guidance [22].

In the process of IMPD preparation the prime challenge is to establish quality specifications for radiopharmaceutical precursors. They are supposed to comprise a set of tests that are necessary to confirm identity, purity and strength of the drug substance. Issues under consideration are the definition of release criteria, analytical procedures and especially their validation. Main references to address these issues are the European Pharmacopeia and guidance provided by the International Conference

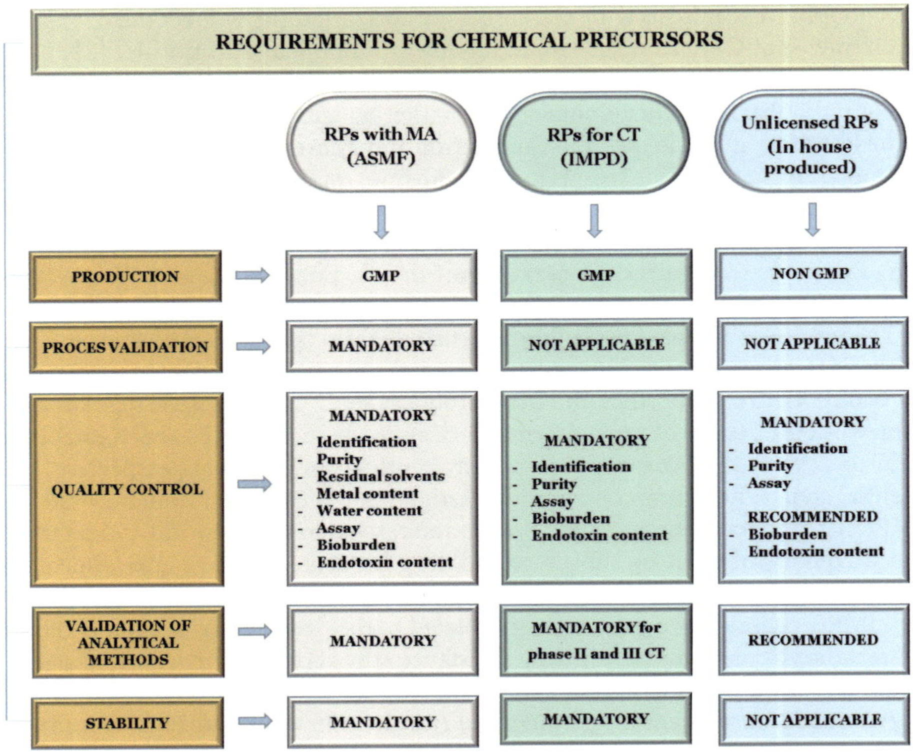

Figure 2.
Requirements for chemical precursors used in preparation of radiopharmaceuticals depending on their regulatory status.

on Harmonization (ICH). Ph. Eur. provides general requirements for quality control of radiopharmaceutical precursors, in addition, a number of monographs for individual radiopharmaceuticals and chemical precursors are available in the Ph. Eur.

The use of analytical methods described in the pharmacopeia allows to reduce the work load related to analytical method validation. This does not mean that a pharmacopeia method may be implemented without any preliminary testing and verification. As a minimum, the most critical parameters should be verified, depending on the intended method. If no pharmacopeia monograph exists, analytical methods need to be fully validated. As stated by the general reference document issued by ICH the objective of validation of an analytical procedure is to demonstrate that it is suitable for its intended purpose [23]. To validate an analytical method, the following characteristics may be considered: specificity, accuracy, linearity range, precision (repeatability and intermediate precision), limit of detection (LOD), limit of quantitation (LOQ) and robustness. Recently, recommendations for the validation of analytical methods which are specific for radiopharmaceuticals has been published by EANM [24].

3. Chemical precursors for radiopharmaceutical preparations

Chemical precursors for radiopharmaceutical preparations, are non-radioactive substances obtained by chemical synthesis for combination with a radionuclide in contrast to precursors manufactured using substances of human or animal origin [4].

The quality specification for chemical precursors is built upon three elements: exact methods, test limits and selection of reference standard. Pharmacopeia monographs comprise a set of critical attributes categorized into three subdivisions: identity, tests (related substances, residual solvents, metal catalyst or metal reagent residues, microbial contamination, bacterial endotoxin) and assay of the active substance. To ensure the appropriate quality, reference substances (like primary standards e.g. Ph. Eur. Chemical Reference Substance, CRS, or Pharmaceutical Secondary Standard, PSS) are used as a standard in an assay, identifications, or purity test. CRS or PSS are often characterized and evaluated for its intended purpose by additional procedures other than those used in routine testing [25].

For in-house prepared radiopharmaceuticals the confirmation of the chemical identity and purity of the precursor are the minimum quality control required, in order to qualify the material for subsequent clinical radiolabeling. Additional testing may apply if necessary for the specific process. For example, testing of trace metals content may not be necessary when the material will be subsequently radiolabeled with halogens, but is absolutely critical when the material is intended for labelling with radiometals [26].

To bring a novel radiopharmaceutical into the clinic it is needed that specific quality requirements for the radiopharmaceutical precursor are established, the range of testing would depend on their status and/or intended use. It is worth noting that for Phase I clinical trials full analytical validation is not necessary (only method suitability should be confirmed) [21]. While analytical methods used to evaluate a batch of API for clinical trials may not yet be validated, they should be scientifically sound [27].

There are some specific requirements for the large-sized molecules (e.g. proteins or monoclonal antibodies) as radiopharmaceutical precursors [28]. Monoclonal antibodies are immunoglobulins (Ig) with a defined specificity derived from a monoclonal cell line. Their biological activities are characterized by a specific binding characteristic to a target ligand (e.g. antigen) and they may be generated by recombinant DNA (rDNA) technology, hybridoma technology, B lymphocyte immortalization or other technologies. Generally, when chemical precursors are manufactured using substances of human or animal origin, the requirements of Ph. Eur. chapter 5.1.7. Viral safety [29] and the general monograph Products with risk of transmitting agents of animal spongiform encephalopathies (1483) [30] apply.

Stability testing is part of the chemical precursor's characterization. Detailed requirements for carrying out stability studies are included in the ICH guideline Q1A (R2) [31]. The purpose of stability testing is to provide evidence on how the quality of a substance varies with time under the influence of a variety of environmental factors such as temperature, humidity, and light, and to establish a re-test period and recommended storage conditions. Stability studies should be carried out on at least three batches and include testing parameters of the chemical precursor that are susceptible to changes during storage and may affect quality, safety and efficacy (e.g. chemical purity and/or assay). The validated analytical methods should be used in these tests. For method validation, it is essential to investigate degradation products and establish degradation pathways under stress conditions (e.g. heat, humidity, light, acid/base hydrolysis and oxidation).

4. Peptides as precursors for radiopharmaceutical preparations

4.1 General consideration

Peptides are an emerging class of compounds that have application in theranostics of several diseases, mainly in cancer [32–36]. These chemical precursors are positioned between the classic small organic molecules and the high molecular weight biomolecules. The interest of the scientific community for peptide drugs has been continuously growing. Currently, more than 60 peptide-based pharmaceuticals are marketed, over 150 peptides are in active clinical trials and estimated 500 more are in preclinical stages of development [37, 38]. Chemically, peptides have poly-amino acids structure ranging from 3 to 100 amino acids (less than 10 kDa) linked by a peptide (amide, –CONH–) bond, and are lacking a tertiary structure. From the biological point of view, peptides are important regulators of growth and cellular functions in normal tissue and tumors. They can act as cytokines, chemokines, neurotransmitters, hormones and growth factors. Generally, they offer many advantages over other groups for radiopharmaceutical applications. Peptides demonstrate high receptor specificity and selectivity, as well as binding affinity, good tissue penetration and favorable pharmacokinetic profiles. Most of them is characterized by low toxicity and immunogenicity [39, 40]. Their compact size results in rapid targeting and blood clearance. As a consequence low nonspecific uptake in non-targeted tissues and high target-to-background ratios are achieved. Moreover, peptides can be easily chemically synthesized in high purity, modified and stabilized to obtain optimized pharmacokinetic parameters. These all attributes together with ability to attach different chelating agents, prosthetic group and availability of various bioconjugation techniques make peptides an important target platform for theranostic radiopharmaceuticals [41, 42].

Peptide-based radiopharmaceuticals were introduced into the clinic more than three decades ago [43]. Since that time, several theranostic radioligand platforms are used for diagnosis and peptide receptor radionuclide therapy (PRRT) of different cancer types. In this concept, peptide analogs directed against somatostatin receptors (SSTR) play a crucial role [44]. The most prominent example of the theranostic pair of radiolabeled peptides are DOTA-conjugated SSTR agonist DOTA-(D-Phe^1, Tyr^3, Thr^8)-octreotate (DOTA-TATE) labeled with ^{68}Ga and ^{177}Lu (**Figure 3**). The marketing authorization of NETSPOT® ([^{68}Ga]Ga-DOTATATE) in 2016 and LUTATHERA® ([^{177}Lu]Lu-DOTATATE) in early 2018 [45] encouraged the research in this field to develop improved radiolabeled peptides targeting other receptor/antigen families, exemplified by the prostate specific membrane antigen (PSMA) [46], gastrin-releasing peptide receptor (GRPr) [47] and cholecystokinin-2 receptor (CCK_2R) [48, 49]. Some of these peptides are currently under clinical investigation.

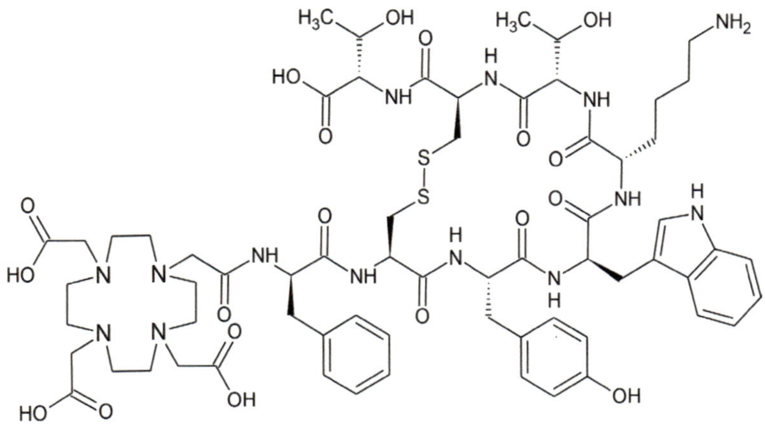

Figure 3.
Structure of DOTA-TATE for labelling with theranostics pair of radionuclides: Gallium-68 (^{68}Ga) and lutetium-177 (^{177}Lu).

4.2 Quality aspects

Peptides as precursors for radiopharmaceutical preparations, similarly to other chemical precursors, require adequate specification as a part of their quality assurance in order to demonstrate the safety and efficacy of the final radiopharmaceutical preparation. Currently, no individual pharmacopeia monograph of peptide used as radiopharmaceutical precursors is available. Thus, the quality specification should be established according to the general requirements [4, 50]. Herein, we provide an overview of recommended methods and test limits for the characterization of peptides. The set of analytical procedures that need to be considered is presented in **Table 1**. However, it should be noted that new analytical methods and modifications to existing ones are continuously being developed and should be utilized where appropriate.

Parameters	Typical methods	Typical acceptance criteria
Characters		
- Appearance/color	Visual inspection	White or almost white powder
- Solubility	Visual inspection	Solubility in water, ethanol and dilute acid or alkali
Identification		
- Active moiety	RP-HPLC-UV	Retention time *versus* reference
	MS or	Mass spectrum *versus* reference
	NMR	NMR spectrum *versus* reference
	IR	IR spectrum *versus* reference
	AAA (GC)	AA: theoretical content ±20%
Purity tests		
- Related substances	HPLC-UV	Individual, unidentified: < 2.0% Total: ≤ 3.0%
- Residual solvents	(Headspace) GC	Acetonitrile: ≤ 0.5%
- Residual metals	AAS/ICP-AES/ICP-MS	Pt, Pd, Ir, Rh, Ru, Os, Mo, Ni, Cr, V, Pb, Hg, Cd, Tl: ≤ 0.01%
- Residual reagents	HPLC-UV/IC/GC	Trifluoracetic acid: ≤ 1.0%*
Counter-ion content	HPLC-UV/IC/GC	Acetic acid: target ±5% Trifluoracetic acid: target ±5%
Water content	Karl-Fisher	≤ 10.0%
Assay (net peptide content)	RP-HPLC-UV or CHN	≥ 75.0%
Bioburden	TAMC plate count	≤ 10^3 CFU/g for bulk ≤ 10^2 CFU per container
	TYMC plate count	≤ 10^2 CFU/g for bulk ≤ 10^1 CFU per container
Bacterial endotoxins	Gel-clot	≤ 100 IU/g for bulk ≤ 10 IU per container

**The residual TFA content is determined when AcOH or HCl are used as counter-ions.*

Table 1.
Summary of the recommended quality parameters for peptides used as radiopharmaceutical precursors.

4.2.1 Appearance

The preliminary quality evaluation of peptides is based on the visual inspection of the appearance/color and solubility. This parameter is given only for information, it is not a requirement in a strict sense. If any of the characteristics change during storage, this change should be investigated and appropriate action taken. A typical description of peptide appearance is: white to almost white, freeze-dried powder and solubility is stated in water, ethanol and dilute solutions of acids and alkali [38, 51].

4.2.2 Identification

According to the ICH Q6A guideline [25] identification testing should allow to discriminate between compounds of closely related structure which are likely to be present (e.g. peptides with altered sequences or functional groups that may be formed during the synthesis). The identification test should include combination of different procedures (mostly two) and should be specific and unequivocal. Several techniques are currently in use for confirmation of peptide identity: HPLC-UV, nuclear magnetic resonance spectrometry (NMR), mass spectrometry (MS), infrared absorption spectrophotometry (IR), amino acid analysis (AAA) or peptide sequencing [51]. The method of choice is typically HPLC-UV based on retention time by comparison with reference standard, since the separation by RP-HPLC is often utilized and the method is widely available. UV detection of peptides is realized at 210–220 nm and 250–290 nm for aromatic side chains of phenylalanine, tyrosine and tryptophan. Identification solely by a chromatographic retention time is not regarded as specific and should be complemented by spectrometric techniques. The NMR spectroscopy is the method that allows to unequivocally define the structure of a peptide in the terms of amino acid composition, sequence and chirality. Identification by NMR spectrometry is usually limited to peptides comprising up to 15 amino acids and requires complex data interpretation. For this reason NMR technique is primarily replaced by mass spectroscopy (MS). This technique provides highly accurate molecular weight information on intact molecules, which is an advantage of MS for peptide identification. The peptide molecular mass is most commonly determined by using the electrospray ionization method (ESI), which occurs through the addition or removal of protons and appears as singly or doubly charged ions. As alternative for the more sophisticated spectroscopic methods, amino acid analysis (AAA) could be considered. This technique involves the hydrolysis of the peptide (usually in acidic conditions) to its individual amino acid residues, followed by chromatographic separation and detection/quantification. The method also enables the determination of the enantiomeric purity with the use of appropriate reference standards. However, this method may not be applicable to peptides containing unnatural amino acids and/or specific chelators. The NMR and AAA as well as peptide sequencing techniques are generally used for characterization of PSS.

In the two recently published papers the identity of DOTA-TATE has been confirmed using suitable instrumental techniques; Sikora et al. [52] confirmed the identity of DOTA-TATE using three different methods: MS, IR and HPLC. Similarly, in the work by Raheem at al [53] the final product was analyzed using high resolution mass spectrometry for identification and analytical HPLC for purification; it was detected via analytical HPLC at a retention time of 9.52 min and detected by HRMS-ESI (calc m/z for $[(\text{DOTA-TATE} + 2\text{H})/2]^{+}$: 718.3028, found: 718.3046 with −0.1144 ppm error).

In our experience ESI-MS in positive ionization mode was used to confirmed whether the masses of ions at m/z 1435.6 ± 1.0 $[M + H]^{+}$ and 718.3 ± 1.0 $[M + 2H]^{2+}$

correspond to the monoisotopic mass of peptide [M] as presented in **Figure 4**. DOTA-TATE PSS was used as reference in IR analysis. Also a gradient HPLC-UV (220 nm) served as identity test of DOTA-TATE by comparison with the reference standard (Rt ± 5.0%). The same HPLC method was used for determination of peptide purity and assay. The representative HPLC chromatograms of DOTA-TATE and DOTA-TATE PSS are given in **Figure 5**.

4.2.3 Related substances

Peptides are usually chemically synthesized using solid-phase peptide synthesis (SPPS) [54]. In this multi-stage process, amino acids are linked to each other during individual coupling steps, thus constructing the desired peptide sequence. This occurs when the carboxylic end of the sequence is covalently attached to a solid support matrix. The complexity of the peptide production process results in a greater diversity of potential impurities. Heterogenicity of the impurity profile is observed

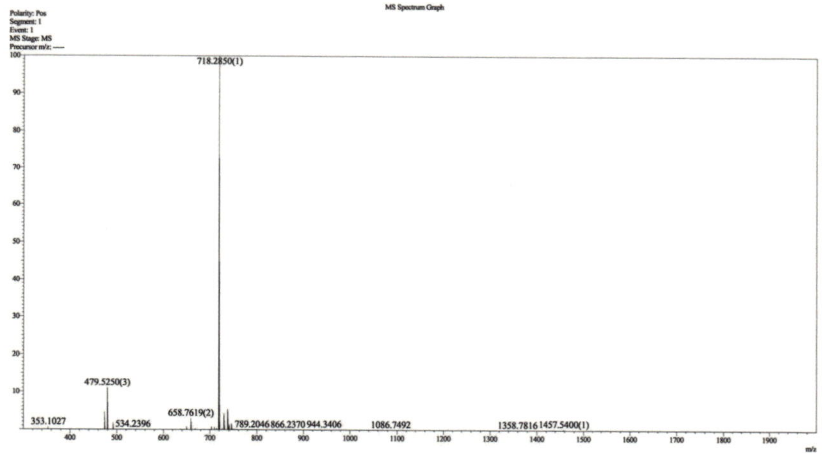

Figure 4.
ESI-MS spectrum for DOTA-TATE.

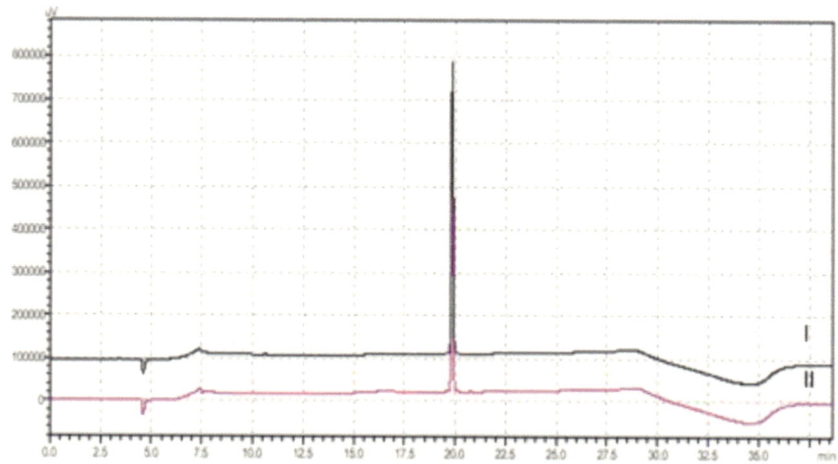

Figure 5.
HPLC-UV (220 nm) chromatograms of (I) DOTA-TATE Rt = 19.831 min and (II) DOTA-TATE PSS Rt = 19,936 min. HPLC method: Luna C18(2) column; Mobile phase - A: water with 0.1% TFA, B: Acetonitrile with 0.1% TFA; gradient profile – From 0 to 25 min: 0–50% B; flow - 0.8 mL/min, oven temperature - 30°C.

even among peptides manufactured by the same synthetic route. The impurities can originate from raw materials, the manufacturing process, degradation or may be formed during storage. Although protecting groups, scavengers or activated functional groups are used to prevent undesired side-chain reactions the peptide manufacturing process leads to formation of closely related impurities. The most common impurities are products of racemization, deamidation, amino acid deletion or insertion, acetylation, oxidation, β-elimination, cyclization, reduction and incomplete deprotection [51]. The presence of related peptide impurities is typically determined using gradient reversed-phase HPLC method with UV detection, because of its selectivity, high sensitivity, low limit of detection, quantification and robustness. The developed HPLC method should allow sufficient separation of potential impurities from manufacturing process as well as degradation products. The acceptance criteria for related substances according to the Ph. Eur. General Monograph 2902 [4] are presented in **Table 2**.

Specific thresholds should be applied for impurities known to be unusually potent or to produce toxic or unacceptable pharmacological effects.

4.2.4 Metallic impurities

The presence of inorganic impurity should also be considered, in particular when radiolabeling of the peptide with radiometals is concerned. According to the Ph. Eur. general monograph (2902), the metal residues in peptides should be determined if the manufacturing process is known or suspected to lead to its presence, e.g. due to the use of specific metal catalyst (e.g. Pd) or metal containing reagents. The content for each of the following metals: Pt, Pd, Ir, Rh, Ru, Os, Mo, Ni, Cr, V, Pb, Hg, Cd, Tl in the peptide precursors are limited to 0.01%. The metal impurities are typically examined using atomic absorption spectrometry (AAS), inductively coupled plasma with atomic emission spectrometry detection (ICP-AES) or mass spectrometry detection (ICP-MS) techniques. Determination of residual metals in peptides can be crucial for precursors intended for radiometal labeling [55]. It has been proven that the presence of certain metals can significantly affect the labeling efficiency through competitive chelation.

4.2.5 Residual solvents

In addition to related substances the residual solvents are required to be examined as impurities in peptide precursors. Residual solvents in pharmaceuticals are defined as organic volatile chemicals that are used in the manufacturing process. The solvents are not completely removed by practical manufacturing techniques (e.g. lyophilization process). General guidelines established by the ICH divide solvents into three classes [56]. The Class 1 solvents should not be used in the final step of the manufacturing process of chemical precursors, because of toxicity and environmental impact. The use of the Class 2 solvents should be limited due to potential toxicity and Class 3 solvents are regarded as posing a lower risk to human

Reporting threshold	0.2 per cent
Identification threshold	2.0 per cent
Total unspecified impurities	Maximum 3.0 per cent

Table 2.
Acceptance criteria for related substances [4].

health. Based on the permitted daily exposure (PDE), Class 2 and 3 solvents are limited to 0.5%. Residual solvents are typically determined using chromatographic techniques such as gas chromatography (GC) coupled with static headspace sampling. Many solvents are usually used in the peptides synthetic process. However, as the advantage of the SPPS and lyophilization process, the most frequently detected solvent is only acetonitrile (Class 2 solvent), used as the component of the mobile phase in the final purification process by preparative HPLC.

4.2.6 Counter-ion content

Synthetic peptides usually contain counter-ions on protonated amino functional groups (N-terminus, Arg, His, Lys, etc.). The presence of counter-ions such as acetate, chloride or trifluoroacetate results from the peptide post synthetic cleavage and/or purification process. Depending on the peptide sequence they reduce the net peptide content by 5 to 25%, but are not considered as impurity. Radiopharmaceutical preparations for diagnostic or therapeutic purposes are based on the net peptide content and thus the amount of residual counter-ions needs to be assessed. To determine counter-ion amounts different method are being used such as: GC, HPLC-UV or ion chromatography (IC). Trifluoroacetic acid (TFA) determined by IC at the level of ca. 20% in DOTA-TATE [52], corresponded to three TFA molecules associated to single peptide molecule. TFA is commonly used as a chemical reagent to remove residual protecting groups during purification of peptides and also as a mobile-phase modifier in a reversed-phase chromatography. Therefore, when the counter-ion finally is AcOH or HCl, determination of the TFA residual content is mandatory.

4.2.7 Water content

In order demonstrate a lot-to-lot consistency the test for water content (residual moisture remaining from the lyophilization process) should be also performed. This parameter may affect the stability of the peptide. For residual water Karl-Fischer titration method as well as GC method with thermal conductivity detector (TCD) [57] are commonly used and water content is limited to max. 10%.

4.2.8 Assay

Generally, assay is defined as a net peptide content. The lyophilized peptide contains also water, counter ions and residual solvents. The net peptide content is referred to percentage of peptide material in the lyophilized peptide. According to ICH guideline Q6A, a specific stability-indicating procedure should be included in the specifications to determine the content of the drug substance. There are two main approaches to determine net peptide content. The first method is a relative assay against a well-defined chemical reference substance, performed using comparative chromatographic procedures. Usually the same RP-HPLC method is used for both assay, identification and related substances. The second approach is an absolute assays involving a functional group (e.g. AAA or titration methods) or a nitrogen content analysis. The nitrogen content is determined from the results of elemental analysis CHN. The calculation of the net peptide content is based on the relation between determined %N to the theoretical content in the peptide structure. For example, this method was used to DOTA-TATE assay determination. Peptide content calculated from elemental analysis was ca. 78.0%, which was in agreement with the generally accepted limit ≥75% [52].

4.2.9 Microbiological assays

The presence of microorganisms may affect the stability of drug substances due to their propensity to degrade/metabolize peptides. Microbiological examinations involve the bioburden control (Ph. Eur 2.6.12) and content of bacterial endotoxins (Ph Eur. 2.6.14). The microbial enumeration tests for total aerobic microbial counts (TAMC) and total yeast and mold counts (TYMC) must adhere to the acceptance criteria of 10^3 CFU/g and 10^2 CFU/g for bulk material and 10^2 CFU/g and 10^1 CFU per container for chemical precursors packed in single and multi-dose containers, respectively. Bacterial endotoxin can be determined by the gel-clot or photometric methods (turbidimetric and chromogenic techniques) and acceptance criteria are limited to a maximum 100 IU/g for bulk material or maximum 10 IU per container for chemical precursors packed in single-dose and multidose containers.

5. Radionuclide precursors

Radionuclide precursors are offered as solutions for radiolabeling with MA, they are also locally produced for the in-house preparation of radiopharmaceuticals. There is an ongoing debate whether radionuclide precursors always have to be considered as medicinal product, or also can be provided as a starting material [58]. Unlike for chemical precursors for radiopharmaceutical preparation, up to date there is no monograph in the Ph. Eur. that sets out general requirements for radionuclide precursors. This is due to the fact that the quality requirements for radionuclides used to obtain diagnostic and therapeutic preparations are highly varying and depend on the irradiation route and chemical processing involved, which mainly affect the parameters of radionuclide purity or specific activity.

However, there are several individual Ph. Eur. monographs for radionuclide precursors. Two of these concern radionuclide precursors used to prepare radiopharmaceuticals for therapeutic use. These are: *Lutetium (^{177}Lu) solution for radiolabelling* (mon. 2798) [59] and *Yttrium (^{90}Y) chloride solution for radiolabelling* (mon. 2803) [60]. There are also six monographs published for radionuclide precursors for preparation of diagnostic radiopharmaceuticals: Fluoride (^{18}F) solution for radiolabelling (mon. 2390) [61], Sodium iodide (^{123}I) solution for radiolabelling (mon. 2314) [62], Sodium iodide (^{131}I) solution for radiolabelling (mon. 2121) [63], Indium (^{111}In) chloride solution (mon. 1227) [64] and Gallium (^{68}Ga) chloride solution for radiolabelling (mon. 2464) [65] and a newly published monograph for Gallium (^{68}Ga) chloride (accelerator-produced) solution for radiolabelling (mon. 3109) [66].

Focusing attention on theranostic radiopharmaceuticals, herein the quality requirements only for metallic radionuclide precursors used in diagnostics and therapy are compared. **Table 3** shows the exemplary quality requirements for radionuclide precursor for therapeutic use (^{177}Lu) and a matching radionuclide precursor for diagnostic use (^{68}Ga).

Comparing the requirements of these two monographs there are apparently large differences in numerical values seen, especially for metal ion content and radiochemical purity. However, when the radioactivity of these radionuclides (different for therapeutic or diagnostic use) is considered, there are basically no differences in quality requirements for both radionuclides. This can be demonstrated on the example of the DOTA-TATE preparations with ^{177}Lu and ^{68}Ga. For therapy 7.4 GBq of [^{177}Lu]Lu-DOTA-TATE is used and this preparation contains ca. 0.2 mg of DOTA-TATE. Typical dose of [^{68}Ga]Ga-DOTA-TATE is 200 MBq and the ligand content in the preparation should not exceed 0.05 mg. Therefore, when analyzing the limit of metallic impurities, e.g. Zn in the radionuclide precursor,

Lutetium (^{177}Lu) solution for radiolabelling (Ph. Eur. 2798 [59])	**Gallium (^{68}Ga) chloride solution for radiolabelling (Ph. Eur. 2464 [60])**
pH: 1.0 to 2.0, using a pH indicator strip R.	*pH:* maximum 2, using a pH indicator strip R.
Lutetium: Inductively coupled plasma-atomic emission spectrometry (2.2.57), for determination of specific radioactivity. *Copper:* maximum 1.0 μg/GBq *Iron:* maximum 0.5 μg/GBq *Lead:* maximum 0.5 μg/GBq *Zinc:* maximum 1.0 μg/GBq	*Iron:* maximum 10 μg/GBq *Zinc:* maximum 10 μg/GBq
RADIONUCLIDIC PURITY *Lutetium-177*: minimum 99.9 per cent of the total radioactivity. Gamma-ray spectrometry. *Results*: - the total radioactivity due to ytterbium-175 (impurity B) is not more than 0.1 per cent; – the total radioactivity due to lutetium-177 m (impurity A) is not more than 0.07 per cent; – the total radioactivity due to radionuclidic impurities other than A and B is not more than 0.01 per cent.	RADIONUCLIDIC PURITY *Gallium-68:* minimum 99.9 per cent of the total radioactivity. A. Gamma-ray spectrometry. *Limit*: peaks in the gamma-ray spectrum corresponding to photons with an energy different from 0.511 MeV, 1.077 MeV, 1.022 MeV and 1.883 MeV represent not more than 0.1 per cent of the total radioactivity. B. Germanium-68 and gamma-ray-emitting impurities. Gamma-ray spectrometry. *Result*: the total radioactivity due to germanium-68 and gamma-ray-emitting impurities is not more than 0.001 per cent.
RADIOCHEMICAL PURITY *[^{177}Lu]lutetium(III) ion*: minimum 99 per cent of the total radioactivity due to lutetium-177.	RADIOCHEMICAL PURITY *[^{68}Ga]gallium(III) ion*: minimum 95 per cent of the total radioactivity due to gallium-68.
Bacterial endotoxins (2.6.14): less than 175 IU/V, V being the maximum volume to be used for the preparation of a single patient dose, if intended for use in the manufacture of parenteral preparations without a further appropriate procedure for the removal of bacterial endotoxins.	*Bacterial endotoxins (2.6.14):* less than 175 IU/V, V being the maximum volume to be used for the preparation of a single patient dose, if intended for use in the manufacture of parenteral preparations without a further appropriate procedure for the removal of bacterial endotoxins.
Sterility: If intended for use in the manufacture of parenteral preparations without a further appropriate sterilization procedure, it complies with the test for sterility prescribed in the mon. 0125. The preparation may be released for use before completion of the test.	

Table 3.
Comparison of Ph. Eur. requirements for selected radionuclide precursors.

similar values are obtained in both cases, i.e. maximum 37 ng and 40 ng per microgram of DOTA-TATE for lutetium-177 and gallium-68, respectively.

When the radiochemical purity is compared, the higher limit of permissible other forms of diagnostic radionuclide ([^{68}Ga]gallium(III) ion: minimum 95%) than for the therapeutic radionuclide ([^{177}Lu]Lutetium(III) ion: minimum 99%) does not result in a higher risk to the patient. Thus, 5% of other forms of a trivalent gallium-68 ion may result in the deposit of 10 MBq of this radionuclide in undesirable chemical form in non-target organs, while for 1% lutetium-177 it is as much as 74 MBq of uncontrolled chemical form. However, it must be noted that a stricter limit for the latter radionuclide is difficult to achieve due to the limitations of the analytical methods, which are characterized by an approximate 1% uncertainty of determination.

Bearing in mind that the differences in the profile of radionuclide contamination depend on the radionuclide production process [67], it is unlikely that uniform quality requirements for radionuclide precursors will be set in numerical terms. Each radionuclide precursor should be evaluated on a case-by-case basis, taking into account the physical characteristics of the radionuclide, its mode of irradiation and chemical processing as well as the envisaged clinical use and the dose planned for administration to the patient. This is clearly reflected in monographs referred in this Chapter. The monograph for ^{177}Lu [59] applies to both the direct and indirect production routes of ^{177}Lu in nuclear reactors and covers all quality aspects regardless the different specific radioactivity and impurity profiles. The decision is left to the producer of the final radiopharmaceutical preparation to use the appropriate solution for radiolabeling. However, the relevant information needs to be stated on the label. This is different in case of ^{68}Ga, there are two different monographs specifying its quality requirements depending whether it's generator [65] or accelerator produced [66]. One can expect that a similar individual approach applies to the future monographs for new theranostic radionuclides, for example ^{47}Sc, which can be either accelerator or reactor produced [68].

6. Conclusion

Are the requirements for radiopharmaceutical precursors overregulated? With the development of new theranostic procedures involving radiopharmaceuticals, there is a need for proper qualitative evaluation of the final radiopharmaceutical preparation and both of the radiopharmaceutical precursors to ensure efficacy and safety of the treatment. An excellent example of the long pathway of a radiopharmaceutical, ^{111}In-CP04, a peptide targeting the cholecystokinin-2 receptor, from the preclinical development over establishing the required pharmaceutical documentation to designing and submitting a clinical trial in patients with Medullary Thyroid Carcinoma, was recently presented [16]. All the quality aspects of CP04 as chemical precursor have been addressed in the IMPD in view of the quality and suitability of the radiolabeled preparation, ^{111}In-CP04, in order to bring it to the clinic.

In this Chapter, the quality requirements applicable to radiopharmaceutical precursors in the context of their regulatory status in Europe were reviewed. EMA and Ph. Eur. provide public standards for manufacture and quality control of these precursors by establishing specifications and acceptance criteria. While in the case of radiopharmaceuticals with MA and CT regulations quite strictly define the quality and documentation requirements, such standards for in-house produced radiopharmaceuticals are still awaited.

DOI: http://dx.doi.org/10.5772/intechopen.95438

Author details

Justyna Pijarowska-Kruszyna[1*], Piotr Garnuszek[1], Clemens Decristoforo[2] and Renata Mikołajczak[1]

1 Radioisotope Centre POLATOM, National Centre for Nuclear Research, Otwock, Poland

2 Department of Nuclear Medicine, Medical University Innsbruck, Austria

*Address all correspondence to: justyna.pijarowska@polatom.pl

References

[1] Lange R, ter Heine R, Decristoforo C. Untangling the web of European regulations for the preparation of unlicensed radiopharmaceuticals: a concise overview and practical guidance for a risk based approach, Nucl Med Commun 2015; 36(5):414. DOI:10.1097/MNM.0000000000000276.

[2] WHO Expert Committee on Specifications for Pharmaceutical Preparation – Radiopharmaceuticals, Final text for addition the International Pharmacopeia, Document QAS/08.262/FINAL, 2008. https://www.who.int/medicines/publications/pharmacopoeia/Radgenmono.pdf

[3] EDQM, General Monograph: 0125, Radiopharmaceutical preparations, European Pharmacopeia, 10th edition, Council of Europe, Strasbourg (2020).

[4] EDQM, Monograph: 2902, Chemical precursor for radiopharmaceutical preparations, European Pharmacopeia, 10th edition, Council of Europe, Strasbourg (2020).

[5] EU Commission, Directive 2001/83/EC of the European Parliament and of the Council of 6 November 2001 on the community code relating to medicinal products for human use. Official Journal of the European Communities, 2004;311:67-128.

[6] EU Commission, Directive 2003/94/EC of 8 October 2003 laying down the principles and guidelines of good manufacturing practice in respect of medicinal products for human use and investigational medicinal products for human use. Official Journal of the European Communities, 2003;262:22-26.

[7] EU Commission, Directive 2004/27/EC of the European Parliament and the Council of 31 March 2004 amending Directive 2001/83/EC on the Community code relating to medicinal products for human use. Official Journal of the European Communities 2004;136:34-57.

[8] EU GMP, Volume 4 Good manufacturing practice (GMP) Guidelines, Annex 3 Manufacture of Radiopharmaceuticals (2008).

[9] EU Commission, Directive 2001/20/EC of the European Parliament and of the Council of 4 April 2001 on the approximation of the laws, regulations and administrative provisions of the Member States relating to the implementation of good clinical practice in the conduct of clinical trials on medicinal products for human use. Official Journal of the European Communities, 2001;121:34-44.

[10] EU Commission, Directive 2005/28/EC of 8 April 2005 laying down principles and detailed guidelines for good clinical practice as regards investigational medicinal products for human use, as well as the requirements for authorization of the manufacturing or importation of such products. Official Journal of the European Communities, 2005;91:13-19.

[11] EU Regulation, No 536/2014 of the European Parliament and of the Council of 16 April 2014 on clinical trials on medicinal products for human use, and repealing Directive 2001/20/EC.

[12] EMA Guidelines on Radiopharmaceuticals. EMEA/CHMP/QWP/306970/2007.

[13] Elsinga P, Todde S, Penuelas I, Meyer G, Farstad B, Faivre-Chauvet A, Mikolajczak R, Westera G, Gmeiner-Stopar T, Decristoforo C. Guidance on current good radiopharmacy practice (cGRPP) for the small-scale preparation of radiopharmaceuticals. Eur J Nucl Med Mol Imaging.

2010;37(5):1049-1062. DOI: 10.1007/s00259-010-1407-3.

[14] Pharmaceutical Inspection Convention Pharmaceutical Inspection Cooperation Scheme. PIC/S guide to good practices for the preparation of medicinal products in healthcare establishments. PE 010-4; 2014.

[15] EDQM, Chapter 5.19. Extemporaneous preparation of radiopharmaceutical preparations, European Pharmacopoeia, 10th edition, Council of Europe, Strasbourg (2020).

[16] Peitl PK, Rangger C, Garnuszek P, Mikolajczak R, Hubalewska-Dydejczyk A, Maina T, Erba P, Decristoforo C. Clinical translation of theranostic radiopharmaceuticals: Current regulatory status and recent examples. 2019;62:673-683. DOI: 10.1002/jlcr.3712.

[17] Verbruggen A, Coenen HH, Deverre JR, Guilloteau D, Langstrom B, Salvadori PA, Halldin C. Guideline to regulations for radiopharmaceuticals in early phase clinical trials in the EU. Eur J Nucl Med Mol Imaging, EANM 2008. DOI: 10.1007/s00259-008-0853-7.

[18] EU Commission Delegated Regulation (EU) 2017/1569 of 23 May 2017 supplementing Regulation (EU) No 536/2014 of the European Parliament and of the Council by specifying principles of and guidelines for good manufacturing practice for investigational medicinal products for human use and arrangements for inspections.

[19] Todde S, Windhorst AD, Behe M, Bormans G, Decristoforo C, Faivre-Chauvet A, Ferrari V, Gee AD, Gulyas B, Halldin C, Peitl PK, Koziorowski J, Mindt TL, Sollini M, Vercouillie J, Ballinger JR, Elsinga PH. EANM guideline for the preparation of an Investigational Medicinal Product Dossier (IMPD). Eur J Nucl Med Mol Imaging. 2014 Nov;41(11):2175-85. doi: 10.1007/s00259-014-2866-8.

[20] Penuelas I, Elsinga PH, The Clinical Translation Process in Europe. In Lewis JS, Windhorst AD, Zeglis BM, editors. Radiopharmaceutical Chemistry. Springer Nature Switzerland AG2019. DOI:10.1007/978-3-319-989471

[21] EMA, Guideline on the requirements for the chemical and pharmaceutical quality documentation concerning investigational medicinal products in clinical trials, EMA/CHMP/QWP/545525/2017.

[22] Todde S, Peitl PK, Elsinga P, Koziorowski J, Ferrari V, Ocak EM, Hjelstuen O, Patt M, Mindt TL, Behe M. Guidance on validation and qualification of processes and operations involving radiopharmaceuticals. EJNMMI Radiopharm Chem. 2017;2(1):8. DOI: 10.1186/s41181-017-0025-9.

[23] ICH guideline Q2(R1), Validation of analytical procedures: text and methodology (2005).

[24] Gillings N, Todde S, Behe M, Decristoforo C, Elsinga P, Ferrari V, Hjelstuen O, Peitl PK, Koziorowski J, Laverman P, Mindt TL, Ocak M, Patt M. EANM guideline on the validation of analytical methods for radiopharmaceuticals. EJNMMI Radiopharm Chem. 2020;12:5(1):7. DOI: 10.1186/s41181-019-0086-z.

[25] ICH Topic Q6A, Specifications: Test Procedures and Acceptance Criteria for New Drug Substances and New Drug Products: Chemical Substances (2000).

[26] IAEA-TECDOC-1856, Quality control in the production of radiopharmaceuticals, IAEA, Vienna, 2018.

[27] ICH Topic Q7, Good Manufacturing Practice for Active Pharmaceutical Ingredients (2000).

[28] EMA, Guideline on development, production, characterization and specification for monoclonal antibodies and related products, EMA/CHMP/BWP/532517/2008.

[29] EDQM, Chapter: 5.1.7, Viral safety, European Pharmacopeia, 10th edition, Council of Europe, Strasbourg (2020).

[30] EDQM, Monograph: 1483, Products with risk of transmitting agents of animal spongiform encephalopathies, European Pharmacopeia, 10th edition, Council of Europe, Strasbourg (2020).

[31] ICH Topic Q1A (R2), Stability Testing of new Drug Substances and Products (2003)

[32] Okarvi SM. Peptide-based radiopharmaceuticals: future tools for diagnostic imaging of cancers and other diseases. Med Res Rev. 2004; 24:357-97. DOI:10.1002/med.20002.

[33] Kaspar AA, Reichert JM. Future directions for peptide therapeutics development. Drug Discov. Today. 2013; 18 (17-18): 807-17. DOI: 10.1016/j.drudis.2013.05.011.

[34] Reubi JC. Peptide receptors as molecular targets for cancer diagnosis and therapy. Endocr Rev. 2003; 24:389-427. DOI: 10.1210/er.2002-0007.

[35] Langer M, Beck-Sickinger AG. Peptides as carrier for tumor diagnosis and treatment. Curr Med Chem Anticancer Agents. 2001; 1:71-93. DOI:10.2174/1568011013354877.

[36] Vlieghe P, Lisowski V, Martinez J, Khrestchatisky M. Synthetic therapeutic peptides: science and market, Drug Discov. Today. 2010; 15:40-56. DOI: 10.1016/j.drudis.2009.10.009.

[37] Lau JL and Dunn MK Therapeutic peptides: historical perspectives, current development trends, and future directions. Bioorg. Med. Chem. 2017;26:2700-2707. DOI: 10.1016/j.bmc.2017.06.052.

[38] Rastogi S, Shatrunajay S, Kalaivani M, Singh GN. Peptide-based therapeutics: quality specifications, regulatory considerations, and prospects. Drug Discov. Today. 2019;24:148-162. DOI:10.1016/j.drudis.2018.10.002220-33.

[39] Fosgerau K, Hoffmann T. Peptide therapeutics: current status and future directions. Drug Discov. Today. 2015;20:122-8. DOI: 10.1016/j.drudis.2014.10.003.

[40] Opalinska M, Hubalewska-Dydejczyk A, Sowa-Staszczak A. Radiolabeled peptides: current and new perspectives, Q J Nucl Med Mol Imag. 2017;61(2):153-67. DOI: 10.23736/S1824-4785.17.02971-5.

[41] Chatalic KLS, Kwekkeboom DJ, de Jong M. Radiopeptides for imaging and therapy: a radiant future. J Nucl Med. 2015;56(12):1809-12. DOI: 10.2967/jnumed.115.161158.

[42] Fani M, Maecke HR, Okarvi SM. Radiolabeled Peptides: Valuable Tools for the Detection and Treatment of Cancer. Theranostics 2012; 2(5):481-501. DOI:10.7150/thno.4024.

[43] Krenning EP, Bakker WH, Breeman WA, Koper JW, Kooij PP, Ausema L, et al. Localisation of endocrine-related tumours with radioiodinated an-alogue of somatostatin. Lancet. 1989;1:242-4. DOI: 10.1016/s0140-6736(89)91258-0.

[44] Eychenne R, Bouvry C, Bourgeois M, Loyer P, Benoist E, Lepareur N. Overview of Radiolabeled Somatostatin Analogs for Cancer Imaging and Therapy. Molecules. 2020;25(17):4012. DOI:10.3390/molecules25174012.

[45] Ballinger JR. Theranostic radiophar maceuticals:established agents in current use. Br J Radiol. 2018;91:20170969. DOI:10.1259/bjr20170969.

[46] Virgolini I, Decristoforo C, Haug A, Fanti S, Uprimny C. Current status of theranostics in prostate cancer. Eur J Nucl Med Mol Imaging. 2018;45(3):471-495. DOI:10.1007/s00259-017-3882-2.

[47] Nock BA, Kaloudi A, Lymperis E, Giarika A, Kulkarni HR, Klette I, Singh A, Krenning EP, de Jong M, Maina T, Baum RP. Theranostic perspectives in prostate cancer with the gastrin-releasing peptide receptor antagonist NeoBOMB1: preclinical and first clinical results. J Nucl Med. 2017;58:75-80. DOI: 10.2967/jnumed.116.178889.

[48] Maina T, Konijnenberg MW, KolencPeitl P, et al. Preclinical pharmacokinetics, biodistribution, radiation dosimetry and toxicity studies required for regulatory approval of a phase I clinical trial with (111)In-CP04 in medullary thyroid carcinoma patients. Eur J Pharm Sci. 2016;91:236-242. DOI:10.1016/j.ejps.2016.05.011.

[49] Uprimny C, von Guggenberg E, Svirydenka A. et al. Comparison of PET/CT imaging with [^{18}F]FDOPA and cholecystokinin-2 receptor targeting [^{68}Ga]Ga-DOTA-MGS5 in a patient with advanced medullary thyroid carcinoma. Eur J Nucl Med Mol Imaging (2020). DOI:10.1007/s00259-020-04963-z.

[50] EDQM, Monograph: 2034, Substances for pharmaceutical use, European Pharmacopeia, 10th edition, Council of Europe, Strasbourg (2020).

[51] Vergote V, Burvenich C, Van de Wiele C, De Spiegeleer B, Quality specifications for peptide drugs: a regulatory pharmaceutical approach. J. Peptide Sci. 2009;15: 697-7. DOI:10.1002/psc.1167.

[52] Sikora AE, Maurin M, Jaron A, Pijarowska-Kruszyna J, Kordowski L, Garnuszek P. Optimization of microwave assisted solid -phase synthesis of octreotate peptide and coupling with protected bifunctional chelator DOTA(tBu)3. Acta Poloniae Pharmaceutica - Drug Research,. 2020;77(4):589-600. DOI: 10.32383/appdr/124745.

[53] Raheem SJ, Schmidt BW, Solomon VR, Salih AK and Price EW. Ultrasonic-Assisted Solid-Phase Peptide Synthesis of DOTA-TATE and DOTA-linker-TATE Derivatives as a Simple and Low-Cost Method for the Facile Synthesis of Chelator–Peptide Conjugates. Bioconjugate Chem. 2020; DOI:10.1021/acs.bioconjchem.0c00325.

[54] Merrifield RB, Solid phase peptide synthesis - Synthesis of a tetrapeptide, J. Am. Chem. Soc. 1963; 85:2149-2154. DOI: 10.1021/ja00897a025.

[55] Asti M, Tegoni M, Farioli D, Iori M, Guidotti C, Cutler CS, Mayer P, Versari A, Salvo D. Influence of cations on the complexation yield of DOTATATE with yttrium and lutetium: a perspective study for enhancing the ^{90}Y and ^{177}Lu labeling conditions. Nucl Med Biol. 2012;39(4):509-17. DOI: 10.1016/j.nucmedbio.2011.10.015.

[56] ICH guideline Q3C (R6) on impurities: guideline for residual solvents (2016).

[57] Nußbaum R, Lischke D, Paxmann H. et al. Quantitative GC determination of water in small samples. Chromatographia 2000;51:119-121. DOI: 10.1007/BF02490705.

[58] Neels O, Patt M, Decristoforo C. Radionuclides: medicinal products or rather starting materials? EJNMMI Radiopharm Chem. 2019;4(1):22. DOI: 10.1186/s41181-019-0074-3.

[59] EDQM, Monograph: 2798, Lutetium (^{177}Lu) solution for radiolabelling, European Pharmacopeia, 10th edition, Council of Europe, Strasbourg (2020).

[60] EDQM, Monograph: 2803, Yttrium (^{90}Y) chloride solution for radiolabelling Yttrium (^{90}Y) chloride solution for radiolabelling European Pharmacopeia, 10th edition, Council of Europe, Strasbourg (2020).

[61] EDQM, Monograph: 2390, Fluoride (^{18}F) solution for radiolabelling, European Pharmacopeia, 10th edition, Council of Europe, Strasbourg (2020).

[62] EDQM, Monograph: 2314, Sodium iodide (^{123}I) solution for radiolabelling, European Pharmacopeia, 10th edition, Council of Europe, Strasbourg (2020).

[63] EDQM, Monograph: 2121, Sodium iodide (^{131}I) solution for radiolabelling, European Pharmacopeia, 10th edition, Council of Europe, Strasbourg (2020).

[64] EDQM, Monograph: 1227, Indium (^{111}In) chloride solution, European Pharmacopeia, 10th edition, Council of Europe, Strasbourg (2020).

[65] EDQM, Monograph: 2464, Gallium (^{68}Ga) chloride solution for radiolabelling, European Pharmacopeia, 10th edition, Council of Europe, Strasbourg (2020).

[66] EDQM, Monograph: 3109, Gallium (^{68}Ga) chloride (accelerator-produced) solution for radiolabelling, European Pharmacopeia, 10th edition, Council of Europe, Strasbourg (2020).

[67] Mikolajczak R, van der Meulen NP, Lapi SE. Radiometals for imaging and theranostics, current production and future perspectives. J Labelled Comp Radiopharm. 2019;62(10):615-634. DOI: 10.1002/jlcr.3770.

[68] Jalilian AR, Gizawy MA, Alliot C, Takacs S, Sudipta Chakarborty, Rovais MRA, Pupillo G, Nagatsu K, Park JH, Khandaker MU, Mikolajczak R, Bilewicz A, Okarvi S, Gagnon K, Al Rayyes AH, Lapi SE, Starovoitova V, Korde A, Osso Jr JA, IAEA Activities on ^{67}Cu, ^{186}Re, ^{47}Sc Theranostic Radionuclides and Radiopharmaceuticals, Curr Radiopharm 2020;13:1. DOI:10.2174/1874471013999200928162322.

Chapter 2

Pretargeted Theranostics

Markus Staudt, Matthias M. Herth
and Christian B.M. Poulie

Abstract

Personalized medicine is becoming an integral part of our healthcare system, in which theranostics play a fundamental role. Nanomedicines such as monoclonal antibodies are a commonly used targeting vector in such approaches due to their outstanding targeting abilities as well as their capabilities to function as drug delivery vehicles. However, the application of nanomedicines in a clinical setting is connected with several challenges. For example, nanomedicines typically possess slow pharmacokinetics in respect to target accumulation and excretion. For targeted radionuclide therapy, this results in high radiation burden to healthy tissue. For drug delivery systems, long circulation and excretion times of the nanomedicine complicate site-specific release approaches and limit as such the usability of these strategies. One way to circumvent these challenges is the use of pretargeting strategies, which allow to separate the accumulation and excretion of nanomedicines from the actual diagnostic or therapeutic application. As such, pretargeting allows to use theranostic concepts utilizing the same nanomedicine and determine the success chances with diagnostic measures before initiating therapy. This chapter will explain the concept of pretargeted theranostics, which pretargeting systems have thus far been developed and compare how these systems performed.

Keywords: radionuclide therapy, PET, SPECT, MRI, radiopharmaceuticals, bispecific antibodies, oligonucleotides, tetrazine/TCO ligation, pretargeting

1. Introduction

Theranostics is a portmanteau of the words therapeutics and diagnostics and is referring to a system were the *modus operandi* of both therapeutic and diagnostic aspects are combined. In this personalized medicine approach, patients are in the first phase non-invasively imaged to identify potential responders to a certain therapy (**Figure 1**) [1]. The ideal theranostic system comprises of a diagnostic and therapeutic agent, which are chemically nearly identical. In reality, the term theranostics is used in a much broader context, i.e. systems that can be used for both diagnostic and therapeutic approaches are also defined as theranostics, even if they differ in their chemical nature [2]. In this chapter, we will discuss theranostics applications mainly in the field of nuclear medicine.

Nanomedicines, especially monoclonal antibodies (mAbs), are finding an ever widespread use in theranostic radionuclide or drug delivery approaches [3]. Unfortunately, nanomedicines typically possess slow target accumulation and excretion times resulting in unwanted and often unacceptably high radiation doses to healthy tissue or limited control in drug release combined with increased systemic toxicity [4]. Pretargeted approaches have the potential to address this challenge by separating the target accumulation process from the diagnostic or therapeutic step.

In pretargeting, a tagged nanomedicine is first administered and allowed to accumulate at its target and excrete from non-targeted tissues over the course of several hours to days. In a second step, a pretargeting agent is administered that bioorthogonally reacts with the tag of the nanomedicine, but is excreted fast from systemic circulation. As such, high and rapid accumulation at the target site can be reached while exposure of the diagnostic or therapeutic component to non-targeted tissues is minimized [5, 6]. Pretargeting is optimally suited for theranostic applications since the pretargeted vector – the nanomedicine – can initially be used for diagnostic purposes and only after having identified the feasibility of the approach, a therapeutic step is initiated (**Figure 2**). Especially in nuclear medicine, such strategy could be highly useful as within the diagnostic phase not only possible responders can be identified, but also the maximum tolerated radiation dose estimated and consequently, on an individual level, best therapeutic efficacy reached (**Figure 1**) [7].

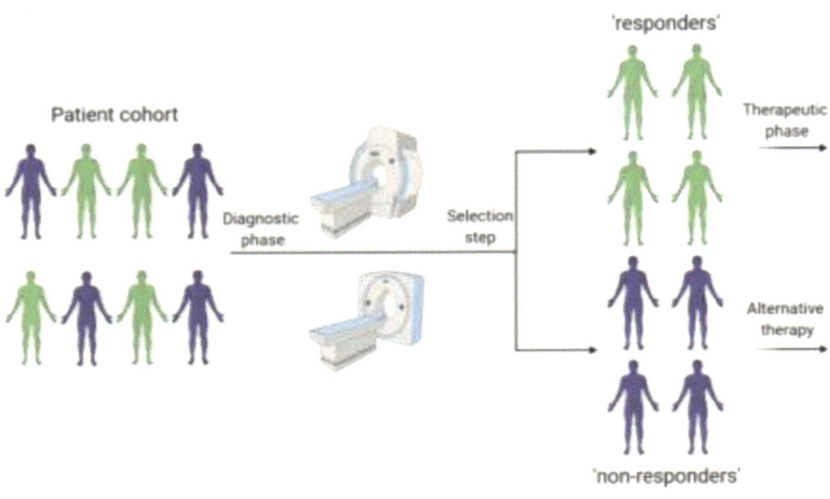

Figure 1.
Personalized medicine. In the diagnostic phase, individuals from the patient cohort that are responding, measured as target accumulation of the nanomedicine, are separated from the non-responders. The responders can move on to the therapeutic phase, whereas for non-responders an alternative treatment form should be applied.

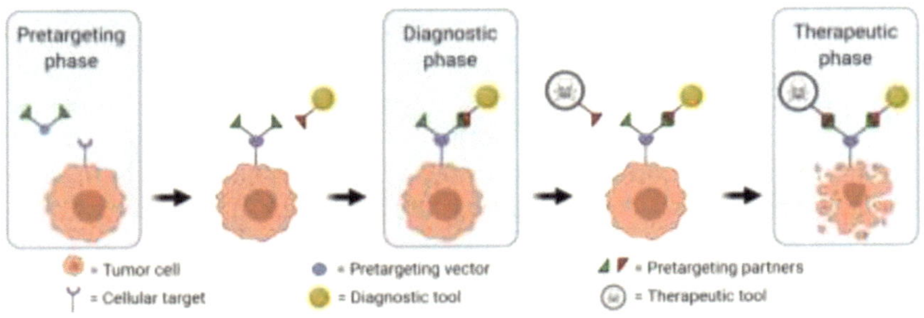

Figure 2.
Simplified schematic overview of a typical pretargeted theranostic strategy.

2. Pretargeted theranostics

2.1 Diagnostic imaging modalities

2.1.1 Positron emission tomography (PET) and single photon emission computed tomography (SPECT)

PET or SPECT are routinely used in the clinic for diagnosis or monitoring of treatment response. Their high sensitivity (the level of detection approaches tracer concentrations of 10^{-12} M) combined with isotopic detection make their clinical applications unmatched [8]. Furthermore, PET can easily be applied for quantitative measurements and as such used to determine e.g. the amount of pretargeting vectors delivered to a specific target. This makes PET especially suited for personalized medicine [9]. One drawback of PET and SPECT is their limited spatial resolution, which lies within the millimeter range [10].

PET and SPECT are dependent on radionuclides that are attached to a specific ligand that is able to target e.g. a specific receptor, enzyme or protein [11]. The choice for the appropriate radionuclide depends on the context and system these diagnostic tools will be used in. For example, if diagnostic radionuclides will be attached to a nanomedicine, longer lived radionuclides are needed, as the biological half-life of the nanomedicines (accumulation or excretion) has to be matched with the physical decay half-life of the radionuclide. Typically, only after several days, nanomedicines display sufficient signal-to-background ratios for imaging purposes [4]. In case of pretargeting, radionuclides with a shorter decay half-life can be used as the good pharmacokinetic profile of small molecules results in fast accumulation and excretion [12]. This allows to use PET radionuclides such as fluorine-18, which is the most frequently used radionuclide within the clinic - due to its unique decay properties [13]. **Table 1** lists several radionuclides that can be used in PET or SPECT imaging.

2.1.2 Fluorescence

While fluorophores are less harmful to tissue in comparison to the use of radionuclides, offer higher temporal and spatial resolution - up to tens of nanometers, fluorophores are majorly disadvantaged by their severely lower tissue penetration of only a few millimeters. This limitation prohibits their use for imaging of deeper lying tissues [14]. Nevertheless, due to their ease of use, fluorescence-based imaging probes are at least within preclinical development a commonly used imaging modality. A list of routinely used fluorophores and their absorption and emission maximum can be found in **Table 2**.

2.1.3 Magnetic resonance imaging (MRI)

MRI is an imaging technique that does not rely on ionizing radiation and therefore has a significantly lower sensitivity (approximately 10^{-4} M) compared to PET or SPECT. However, it results in better spatial resolution [15]. In the context of pretargeted theranostics, a contrasting agent is often added to the pretargeting vector - in order to enhance visibility of the target. The most commonly used contrast agent is gadolinium(III) (Gd^{3+}), in various chelated forms and works by shortening the T_1 (spin–lattice) relaxation time [16]. Another T_1 signal enhancer is manganese(II)

SPECT			PET		
Isotope	$T_{1/2}$ ***(h)***	γ ***(keV)***	***Isotope***	$T_{1/2}$ ***(h)***	β^+ ***(%)***
^{99m}Tc	6.01	140	^{11}C	0.33	99.8
^{111}In	67.3	171 and 245	^{18}F	1.83	96.7
^{123}I	13.3	159	^{64}Cu	12.7	17.5
			^{68}Ga	1.13	89.1
			^{86}Y	14.7	33.0
			^{89}Zr	78.4	22.7
			^{124}I	100.2	22.8

Their corresponding half-lives ($T_{1/2}$) are noted in hours (h). For SPECT radionuclides, the energy of the gamma (γ) photon is noted in keV, for PET radionuclides, their corresponding percent (%) of positron (β^+) decay is noted.

Table 1.
Nuclear properties of common SPECT and PET radionuclides.

Fluorophore	*Absorption maximum [nm]*	*Emission maximum [nm]*
Fluorescein	495	517
AlexaFluor 488	494	519
Cyanine 5	647	665
Cyanine 5.5	672	692
Cyanine 7	753	775
Methylene Blue	665	684
CF-680	681	698
IRDye-800CW	774	789
Indocyanine Green	776	792
Dylight 800	777	794

Table 2.
Absorption and emission maxima of commonly used fluorophores in PBS.

(Mn^{2+}) [17]. Several T_2 (spin–spin) signal enhancers exists, but are less commonly used options. One of these are magnetic nanoparticles (MNP), such as iron oxide or iron/platinum alloys, or alternatively barium(II) (Ba^{2+}) salts. Especially in a theranostic context, decorated MNPs are of great interest as they can simultaneously be used as passive targeting vectors - due to the enhanced permeability and retention (EPR) effect [18].

2.2 Therapy approaches

2.2.1 Radionuclide therapy

Targeted radionuclide therapy approaches have the potential to treat micrometastases and residual tumor tissue remaining after surgical resection – both of which play a major role in the mortality of cancer patients. Currently, only very few radionuclide therapies have found application in clinical practice [19]. This is likely to change in the coming decade, as radionuclide therapy may be more effective than standard therapeutic strategies, e.g. external radiation therapy or state-of-the-art chemotherapy. Two types of radiation can be used in radionuclide-based therapies, namely α- and

Isotope	$T_{1/2}$ *(h)*	*Decay*	*Photon energy (keV)*	*%*
^{67}Cu	61.8	β^-	185	49
^{90}Y	64.6	β^-	1700	0.01
^{131}I	192.5	β^-	364	81
^{177}Lu	159.5	β^-	208	11
^{188}Re	17.0	β^-	155	15
^{211}At	7.2	α	79	21.3
^{213}Bi	0.8	α	440	26
^{212}Pb	10.6	β^- and α	a	a
^{225}Ac	238.1	β^- and α	a	a

Their corresponding half-lives ($T_{1/2}$) are noted in hours, the energy of the photon is noted in keV.
a. Multiple photons, at different energies, are emitted, due to multiple daughter radionuclides.

Table 3.
Nuclear properties of common therapeutic radionuclides.

β^--radiation. In general, α-emitting radionuclides are far more effective due to the significantly higher linear energy transfer (LET) (approx. 100 keV/μm), compared to the much lower LET of β^--emitting radionuclides (approx. 0.2 keV/mm) [4]. However, α-emitters might even be too toxic for many applications.

Just like for the diagnostic case, the choice of radionuclide is highly dependent on the context and system, these radionuclides are used in. With the exception of iodine-131 and astatine-211, all other commonly used radionuclide are radiometals and need to be chelated. As such, these radiopharmaceuticals are typically very polar (**Table 3**). Another factor to be considered is the limited availability of certain radionuclides, such as astatine-211, bismuth-213, lead-212 or actinium-225 [20]. Additionally, lead-212 and actinium-225 have several radioactive daughter nuclides which contribute to radiotoxicity throughout the body when released from the chelator and distributed throughout the body. Due to the high energy released after the first decay event, typically daughter nuclides are released from the chelator and not bound to the chelator any longer [21].

2.2.2 Chemotherapy

Chemotherapy involves the use of highly cytotoxic compounds which are supposed to kill cancer cells more efficiently than healthy cells. In the context of pretargeted approaches, these compounds work in exactly the same manner as in standard chemotherapy approaches, with the crucial difference that they are delivered from the nanomedicine to the target side and then (selectively) released e.g. using click-to-release strategies [22, 23]. A locally increased concentration of the chemotherapeutic is as such achievable, whereas the systemic concentration and its subsequent toxicity is reduced [24]. A few examples of cytotoxic compounds that have been used in conjunction with pretargeted theranostics are paclitaxel, mertansine or doxorubicin [25–27]. However, in theory any cytotoxic drug could be used.

2.3 Pretargeting strategies and their applications as potential Theranostics

2.3.1 Biotin/streptavidin binding

Pretargeting approaches based on the strong, non-covalent interaction between biotin and streptavidin, with a K_d in the order of approximately 10^{-14} M were among the earliest strategies to be successfully applied for pretargeted radioimmuno-imaging and –therapy [4]. In fact, several clinical studies were initiated and are ongoing [28–30]. The strong binding affinity is leveraged by most commonly attaching the tetrameric streptavidin - capable of binding up to four biotins - to a mAb and after sufficient accumulation of this pretargeting vector, radiolabeled biotin is injected as the targeting agent. Despite these successes, reports of this strategy in a theranostic setting are limited. This might be due to the observed increased levels of human anti-streptavidin antibodies, potentially leading to allergic reactions upon subsequent applications [31, 32].

2.3.2 Bispecific antibodies

Bispecific antibodies (bsAb) are artificially constructed immunoconjugates, possessing both an antigen-binding fragment (Fab) - typically targeting an overexpressed receptor on the target cell surface - and an anti-hapten Fab. This allows for targeting the cancer cell while also retaining high affinity to a hapten of choice, which can be used to bind imaging or therapeutic vectors after sufficient accumulation time of the bsAb. Antibody fragments are typically derived from the immunoglobulin G (IgG) antibody, which consists of two Fab sites and a constant fragment crystallizable (Fc) region. Digestion of IgG by pepsin yields the $F(ab')_2$ fragment, which can be further split into two Fab' fragments by mild reduction. Digestion by papain on the other hand yields two Fab fragments. Removal of the two remaining constant domains and relinking them yields fusion proteins called single-chain variable fragment (scFv) (**Figure 3**) [33].

Aniline modified DOTA (DOTA-Bn, **Figure 4**) can act as an efficient chelator for a large variety of (radio)metals and also serve as the hapten. Haptens are small molecular entities that are used to engineer antibodies possessing high affinity to these small molecules, allowing for fragmentation into smaller hapten-binding scFv. In the case of DOTA-Bn, the scFv C825 is capable of binding DOTA-Bn chelated yttrium (Y^{3+}) and lutetium (Lu^{3+}) with picomolar affinity (~15 and 11 pM respectively). This allowed for construction of a IgG-scFv bsAb huA33-C825 (**Figure 4**) targeting GPA33-positive human colorectal cancer cell lines SW1222 [34]. Utilizing this system, SW1222 xenograft bearing mice were subjected to three treatment cycles of pretargeted immunotherapy (PRIT) consisting of injection of bsAb injection, followed by injection of a dextran-hapten clearing agent 24 hours later and injection of [^{177}Lu]Lu-DOTA-Bn after four more hours. SPECT/CT was utilized to follow the treatment, showing high specific tumor uptake (~7% ID/g) and only low uptake (10–15 fold lower) in the liver, the spleen and the kidneys. After three cycles of treatment with 55.5 MBq activity of [^{177}Lu]Lu-DOTA-Bn (at days 7, 14 and 21 after tumor inoculation), 100% histologic cures in 9 of 9 treated

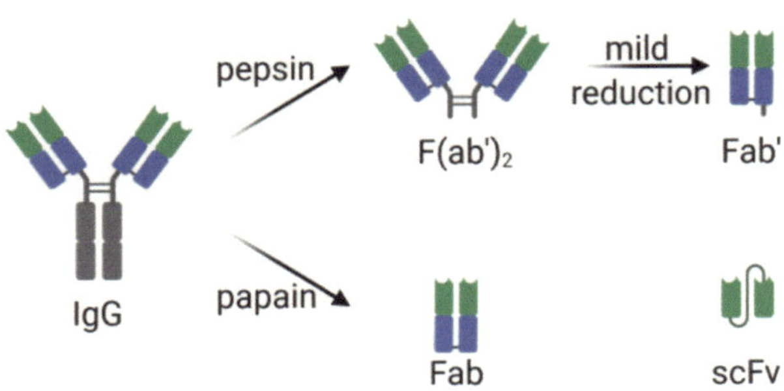

Figure 3.
IgG antibody and its fragments used in the construction of bispecific antibodies.

animals were achieved. Therefore, this approach allows for a theranostic platform with a single radiopharmaceutical entity, allowing for SPECT imaging and providing tumor radiation estimate by changing the amount of radioactivity administered. However, using a therapeutic radionuclide for clinical diagnosis is not optimal since only low amounts can be administered, which often result in insufficient count rates for imaging purposes.

In a similar approach, the food and drug administration (FDA)-approved anti-HER2 antibody trastuzumab, modified with scFv C825 (**Figure 4**), was utilized to target HER2-positive human breast cancer BT-474 xenograft bearing mice [35]. Although internalizing targets like HER2 are normally not suitable for PRIT, it was found that 24 hours post injection of the bsAb around 11% of the initially bound trastuzumab-C825 remained on the cell surface. Using a clearing agent 24 hours after injection of the bsAb, followed by 5.6 MBq of [^{177}Lu]Lu-DOTA-Bn allowed for biodistribution-based dosimetry, showing ~7% ID/g uptake in the tumor with high tumor to blood and kidney ratios (T/B: ~27, T/K: ~10). Given this, the estimated maximum tolerated activity was calculated to be 180 MBq, with blood being the dose-limiting organ. In following therapeutic studies, a single-cycle treatment with 55.5 MBq of [^{177}Lu]Lu-DOTA-Bn was found to lead to 100% complete response (CR) in small tumors up to 30 mm^3, but did not produce a high CR in medium sized tumors (100–400 mm^3). The latter could be successfully treated through three cycle PRIT using 55.5 MBq of [^{177}Lu]Lu-DOTA-Bn, showing 25% complete tumor disappearance and 75% regression to palpitation threshold. Once again, SPECT/CT was used to monitor treatment progression 24 hours p.i. of 55.5 MBq of [^{177}Lu]Lu-DOTA-Bn.

In clinical practice, PET results in better spatial resolution than SPECT. In this regard, a PET tracer based hapten probe was developed [36]. Hapten [^{86}Y]Y-DOTA-Bn was synthesized and used to image a bsAb targeting GPA33-positive cancers [37]. The biodistribution data was in line with the one determined using [^{177}Lu]Lu-DOTA-Bn. Consequently, hapten [^{86}Y]Y-DOTA-Bn can be used as a

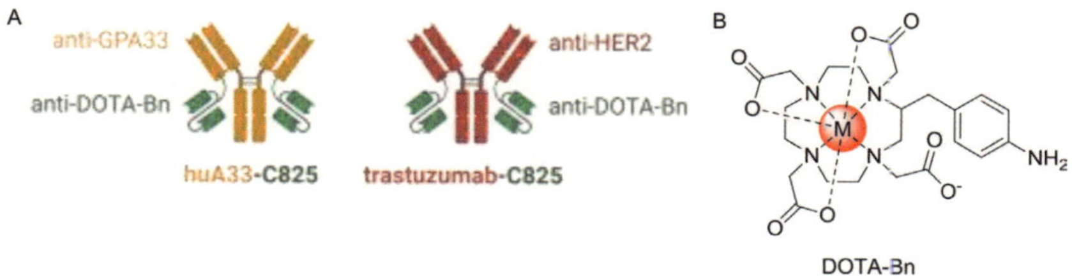

Figure 4.
A: Schematic representation of bsAb huA33–825 and trastuzumab-C825. B: Structure of DOTA-Bn chelating M^{3+}.

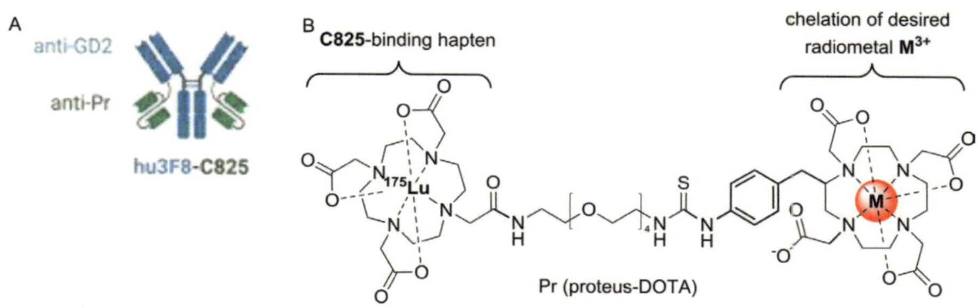

Figure 5.
A: Schematic representation of bsAb hu3F8–C825. B: Structure of proteus-DOTA (Pr) chelating non-radioactive $^{175}Lu^{3+}$ and the radiometal of choice M^{3+}.

surrogate for the ^{177}Lu-labeled derivative. Better diagnostic value and reduced radiation dose should be possible for clinical applications using [^{86}Y]Y-DOTA-Bn.

While the hapten DOTA-Bn allows for straight forward incorporation of yttrium and lutetium, it comes with severe limitations to the modularity of the system as the affinity of the hapten towards scFv C825 varies depending on the chelated metal. This effect was observed in a study on the anti-DOTA antibody scFv –hu3F8-C825 (**Figure 5**), which bound [^{177}Lu]Lu-DOTA-Bn with picomolar affinity, whereas [^{225}Ac]Ac-DOTA-Bn was found to have severely decreased binding [38]. This resulted in a decreased tumor accumulation. To circumvent this problem, a novel construct bearing two DOTA-moieties called proteus-DOTA (Pr, **Figure 5**) was synthesized. By chelating non-radioactive, isotopologic lutetium-175 in one of the DOTA moieties, the construct is able to bind with high affinity to previously utilized scFv C825, while retaining the ability to chelate a radiometal of choice in the second DOTA chelator (**Figure 5**). Using this system, high tumor and relatively low normal tissue accumulation of both [^{111}In]In-Pr and [^{225}Ac]Ac-Pr was achieved. This approach was then successfully employed in a pretargeted therapeutic approach in treating three solid human cancer xenograft models of colorectal cancer (GPA33), breast cancer (HER2), and neuroblastoma (GD2) using the respective anti-tumor/C825 bsAb, followed by injection of a dextran clearing agent after 24 h and four hours later the radiohapten [^{225}Ac]Ac-Pr.

Another promising approach lies in changing the utilized hapten to the small peptidic sequence histamine-succinyl-glycine (HSG). In this respect, the bivalent hapten IMP288 modified with two HSG and DOTA and the trivalent bsAb TF2 were identified to be the most promising pair for clinical translation of this pretargeted system (**Figure 6**) [39]. The trivalent bsAb TF2 was build up through a dock-and-lock approach, linking two anti-carcinoembryonic antigen (CEA) Fabs, binding to the cancers expressing CEA, and one anti-HSG Fab linked through two disulfide bounds (**Figure 6**). This approach allows to label IMP288 with a set of radiometals for both therapeutic and diagnostic purposes. Subsequent preclinical studies in mice bearing CEA-expressing colonic tumors showed very low uptake in normal tissues - apart from the kidneys (~2% ID/g) – and high tumor uptake using PET or SPECT imaging with [^{68}Ga]Ga-IMP288 (~11% ID/G) or [^{111}In]In-IMP288 (~26% ID/G) [40]. These imaging data was successfully used for dose estimations of [^{177}Lu]Lu-IMP288 and [^{213}Bi]Bi-IMP288 [41, 42].

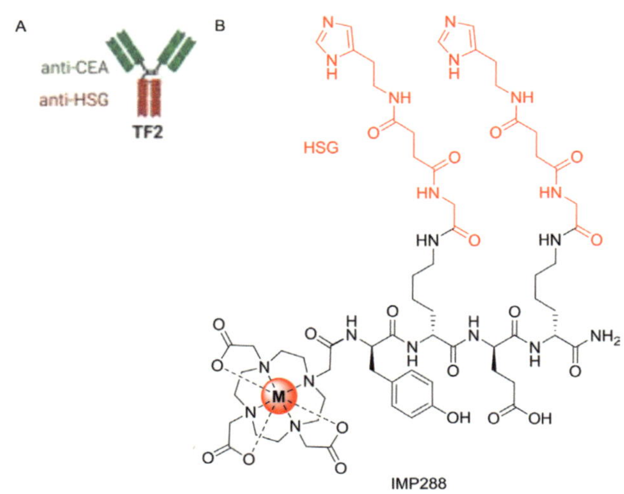

Figure 6.
A: Schematic representation of bsAb TF2. B: Structure of IMP288 chelating M^{3+}.

Given this promising data, the IMP288/TF2 system was translated into the clinic using [^{111}In]In-IMP288 in the imaging cycle for predictive patient-specific dosimetry and [^{177}Lu]Lu-IMP288 as the therapeutic agent. Herein, it was shown, that the treatment of metastatic colorectal cancer patients at activity doses ranging from 2.5 to 7.4 GBq of [^{177}Lu]Lu-IMP288 was safe, but only one of the four planned treatment cycles was carried out since all patients showed progression of the disease, 8 weeks after the first cycle [43]. Also immunogenic responses towards the humanized bsAb TF2 were observed in 11 out of 21 patients. Surprisingly, this immunogenic response was only observed to a very limited degree in one out of eight patients in another study using the same system on advanced lung cancer patients [44].

2.3.3 Oligonucleotides

A more recently employed pretargeting strategy relies on the strong interaction between complementary strands of oligonucleotides. Although unmodified desoxyribonucleic acids (DNAs, **Figure 7**) and ribonucleic acids (RNAs, **Figure 7**) are not suitable for in vivo use due to their rapid degradation by nucleases, recent developments of peptide nucleic acids (PNAs, **Figure 7**) have shown promise in pretargeting. PNAs increase enzymatic stability by replacing the sugar-phosphate backbone of DNAs/RNAs by a pseudo-polypeptidic backbone consisting of a *N*-(2-aminoethyl)-glycine units [45]. PNAs retain Watson-Crick base-pair binding to complementary PNA, DNA or RNA strands. The interaction between PNA/PNA is with greater specificity and binding affinity compared to the corresponding DNA/DNA analogs. A fourth alternative to DNAs, which is stable to enzymatic degredation are phosphorodiamidate morpholino oligomer (morpholinos, **Figure 7**) [46]. Here, the sugar-phosphate moiety is replaced by a methylenemorpholine ring, linked through phosphordiamidate groups.

In a pretargeted study using the PNA-affibody conjugated with $Z_{HER2:342}$-SR-HP1 and a complementary PNA-based DOTA derivative (HP2), the biodistribution patterns of [^{68}Ga]Ga-HP2 and the therapeutic PNA [^{177}Lu]Lu-HP2 were evaluated in SKOV3 xenografts [47]. Overall, quite profound differences in biodistribution between [^{68}Ga]Ga-HP2 (~6% ID/g tumor and ~ 9% kidney accumulation) and [^{177}Lu]Lu-HP2 (~12% ID/g tumor and ~ 8% kidney accumulation) were found, making precise prediction of therapeutic uptake of the latter difficult [48]. This study exemplified that the choice of a theranostic pair, here gallium-68 and lutetium-177, can have an influence on the biodistribution of the labeled radiopharmaceutical. Different stability or altered dipole moments within the chelated structure are some of the possible reasons for this behavior.

2.3.4 Tetrazine/trans-cyclooctene (TCO) ligation

Another strategy for pretargeting involves the covalent bond forming ligation between an 1,2,4,5-tetrazine and a TCO [49]· The reaction is initiated with an enthalpically driven strain release of the inverse electron demand Diels-Alder

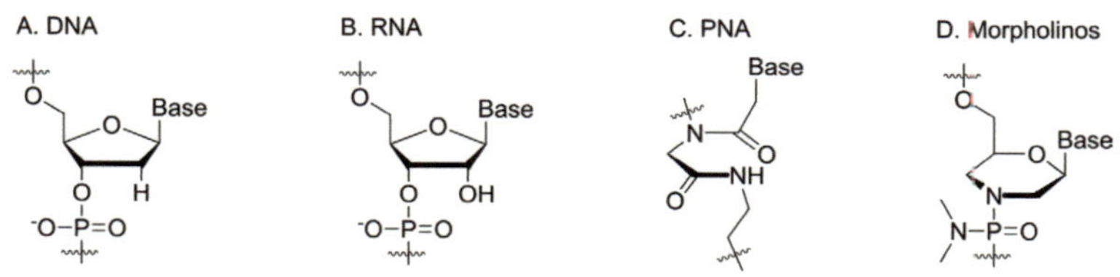

Figure 7.
Structure of DNA, RNA, PNA and morpholino oligonucleotides.

(IEDDA) cycloaddition. The cycloaddition is followed by an entropically driven retro Diels-Alder reaction, in which molecular nitrogen is expelled, making this reaction irreversible (**Figure 8A**) [50]. Variously substituted tetrazines and TCO analogues can be used for this ligation, all differing in their corresponding speed kinetics and in vivo stability. As a general trend, with increasing in vivo stability, a decrease in speed kinetics is observed and vice versa.

The most common approach for pretargeting using the tetrazine ligation is based on TCO-modifications of nanomedicines, which act as pretargeting vectors [51]. These vectors can first be imaged by a tetrazine probe and followed up with a treatment phase, using a therapeutic, tetrazine based probe. For example, the CEA targeting mAb 35A7 was decorated with approximately 3–4 TCO tags and four different [^{177}Lu]-bispyridyl-tetrazine probes used to evaluate the effectiveness of the pretargeted approach. SPECT was used to determine the in vivo biodistribution of the various tracers and gain insights about maximum tolerated dose. The most promising probe was used in a treatment approach and a projected dose of 40 MBq was applied. This resulted in a significant slow-down of tumor progression, for up to 13 days, after which the tumors started to grow again, albeit much slower as compared to the control group [52].

In a similar approach, using a human colorectal carcinoma mouse model, a transmembrane glycoprotein (the A33 antigen) targeting mAb huA33 was decorated with approximately 2–3 TCO tags. Two different tetrazine probes were administered [53]. 24 hours after administration of the huA33-TCO a [^{64}Cu]-H-tetrazine probe was injected and used for diagnostic PET imaging. This was followed by an injection of a [^{177}Lu]-H-tetrazine probe, after an additional 24 hours (48 hours post mAb injection). It was estimated that after the injection of the diagnostic tetrazine, roughly 64% of the TCOs on the mAb were available, for the therapeutic tetrazine probe. This study showed that the same targeting vector can be used for imaging and therapy purposes and as such for real theranostic approaches. The same group also evaluated a ^{67}Cu-labeled H-tetrazine in the same setup for β^-radiotherapy [54]. Within this study, the authors compared the therapeutic effect of pretargeted radioimmunotherapy (PRIT) to conventional radioimmunotherapy (RIT). Even though RIT achieved a comparable survival rate, at lower injected dose, compared to PRIT, it is important to note that PRIT significantly reduced the individual organ dose rates, in comparison to RIT, i.e. the radiation dose to the blood for the PRIT strategy

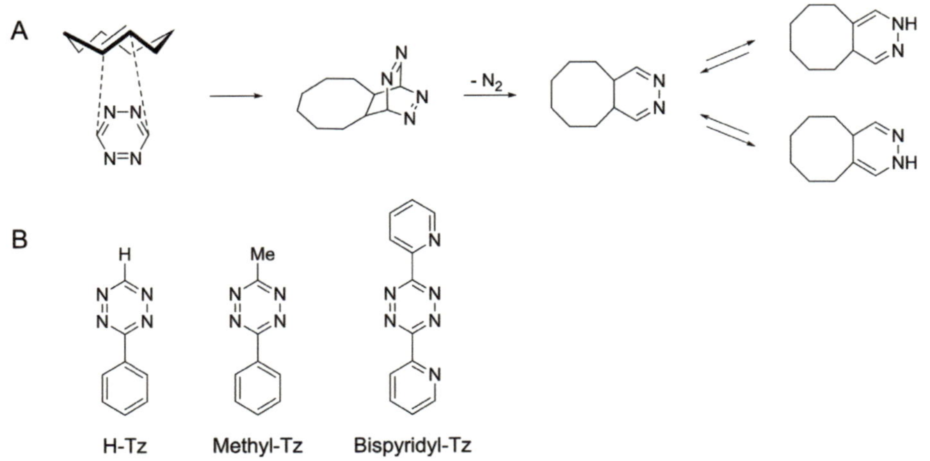

Figure 8.
(A) Mechanism of the tetrazine/TCO ligation. (B) Chemical scaffold of a H-, a methyl- and a bispyridyl-tetrazine.

was 5.9 cGy/MBq, compared to 71.3 cGy/MBq for the RIT strategy, highlighting the main advantage of PRIT over RIT. The authors argued that the PRIT strategy can be further optimized in regards of timing of the dosing regimen, in order to achieve optimal dose rates to the tumor.

In addition to small molecule tetrazine derivatives, also tetrazine functionalized nanocarriers, such as human serum albumin (ALB), can be used as pretargeting vectors. These structures can additionally be modified e.g. with chemotherapeutic agents or fluorophores. Such a strategy was used for trastuzumab, a human epidermal growth factor receptor 2 positive (HER2+) targeting mAb. This mAb was decorated with six TCO moieties and two CF-680 near infrared (NIR) fluorophores [55]. After eight hours, a ALB nanocarrier was injected containing approximately 2–3 paclitaxel molecules, 15 methyl-tetrazines and two DyLight 800 (DL-800) NIR fluorophores. Imaging studies revealed that the tumor uptake was twice as high in mice after two days in the pretargeted group compared to the control group. Also, treated animals only showed a relative increase of tumor volume of 3%, whereas the control group saw an increase of 14%. In another study, eight TCO's were attached to 5D3, a prostate-specific membrane antigen (PSMA) targeting mAb, as well as eight TCO to its F(ab′)2 fragments [56]. Both moieties were additionally decorated with two AlexaFluor 488 (AF-488) fluorophores. ALB was used as the pretargeting agent and possessed 10 methyl-tetrazine handles, two rhodamine fluorophores and approximately 3–4 mertansine molecules, as a therapeutic component. Imaging studies revealed, that the F(ab′)2 fragments internalized faster compared to the whole mAb. Faster internalization is, however, disadvantageous since the internalized targeting vector is not available for the ligation with ALB. This nanocarrier cannot cross the cell membrane. Consequently, less cytotoxic drug can reach its target. No in vivo evaluation of this approach was performed.

Recently, a new click-to-release strategy was described which results in local increased drug concentration and as such increased treatment efficacy. In such an approach, the TCO component acts as a bioorthogonally click partner as well as a drug releasing component. The initial click mechanism is also based on the IEDDA (**Figure 8A**). However, the formed 4,5-dihydropyridazine will partly tautomerize to 1,4-dihydropyridazine which can lead to a release - via a self-immolative cascade reaction - of the chemotherapeutic drug in allylic position (attached e.g. via a carbamate to the TCO) (**Figure 9**). Such a TCO is also called release TCO (rTCO). This click-to-release strategy has also been employed in a theranostic context. For example, in tumor bearing mice expressing the tumor-associated glycoprotein-72 (TAG72), a CC49 diabody – targeting this glycoprotein and side-specifically conjugated to a rTCO decorated with monomethyl auristatin E (MMAE)) – was evaluated [57]. Mice were injected with the diabody 48 prior to injection of an

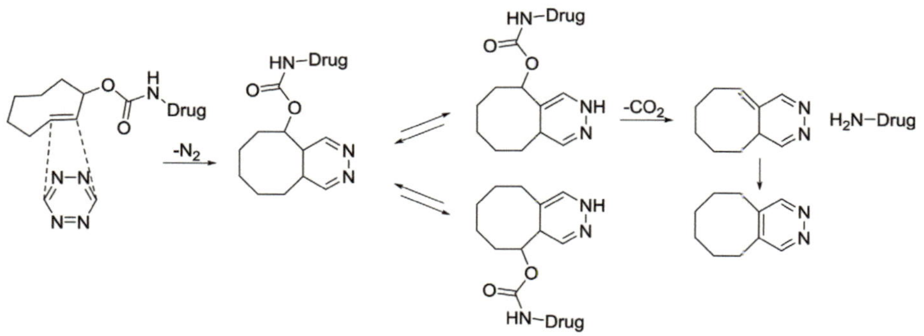

Figure 9.
Mechanism of the click-to-release reaction.

^{111}In-labeled releaser bisalkyl-tetrazine. This set-up allowed to image the release via SPECT. In a different setup, [^{111}In]bispyridyl-tetrazine was used to determine the diabody tumor uptake, as bispyridyl-tetrazines have extremely poor release capabilities for the used rTCO. The gained information was then used to design a treatment study. Four cycles, over a period of two weeks, were used in this study and extended the median survival by 34–39 days. In a different study, a PEGylated hyper-branched polymeric (HBP) nanocarrier was developed bearing rTCOs bound to the drug doxorubicin [58]. In order to achieve a modular approach, HBP was bound to a bsAb, which could selectively interact with PEGs of the HBP with one binding site, whereas the other binding site simultaneously target with the epidermal growth factor receptor (EGFR) or TAG72. A ^{64}Cu-labeled H-tetrazine was used both as the releaser and as an imaging component. This theranostic approach was evaluated in mice bearing MCF7 and MDA-MB-468 tumors. Highest release of doxorubicin was found when the tetrazine was injected 24 hours post nanocarrier injection. Furthermore, better release was observed in non-internalizing targets compared to internalizing targets, as the polar tetrazine was not able to cross the cell membrane.

Lastly, dextran-coated iron oxide MNPs (~25 nm in size) were surface modified with methyl-tetrazines and the NIR fluorophore cyanine5.5 (Cy5.5) [59]. The MNP uptake was monitored by fluorescence, as well as by T_2-weighted MRI. Targeting of these MNP was based on the EPR effect. Conceptually, selective drug release should be induced by a small molecule drug-TCO conjugate which should find the MNP-tetrazine modified targeting vector in vivo and upon reaction release the drug load. Unfortunately, the release was only in vitro, in MDA-MB-231 cells. As such, no real conclusion about the in vivo efficacy can be drawn as well as of the theranostic abilities of the system.

2.3.5 Strain-promoted azide-alkyne cycloaddition (SPAAC)

SPAAC has been applied in pretargeting. The reaction is based on a [3 + 2] cycloaddition between an azide and a strained alkyne (**Figure 10**). Opposed to the copper-catalyzed azide-alkyne cycloaddition (CuAAC), this reaction is metal free and instead entirely entropy driven. Various different constrained alkynes can be used for this biorthogonal reaction, i.e. difluorocyclooctynes (DIFO), bicyclononyne (BCN), dibenzocyclooctynes (DIBO), biarylazacyclooctynone (BARAC), among others. However, the most used alkyne is azadibenzylcyclooctyne (ADIBO/DIBAC), commonly referred to as DBCO. However, the feasibility of the SPAAC appears to be very limited due to its very slow reaction kinetics [60].

2.3.6 Miscellaneous

Besides the previously mentioned strategies, some lesser known and underexplored strategies exist. These are all based on high affinity interactions. One such set of interaction partners is based on the high affinity (~5×10^4 M^{-1}) between β-cyclodextrin, as the host and an adamantine derivative as the guest molecule [61].

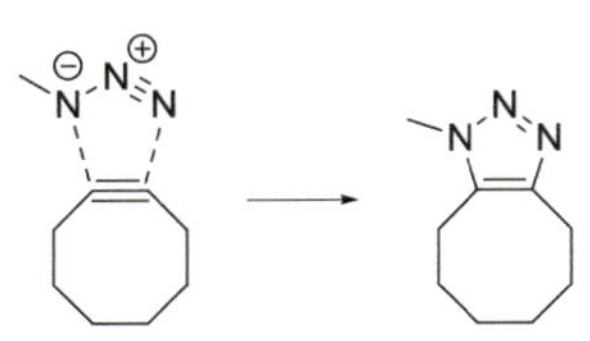

Figure 10.
Mechanism of the strain-promoted azide-alkyne cycloaddition (SPAAC).

This approach has been used in hepatic radioembolization where a macro ALB aggregate (MAA) was decorated with approximately 10^8 adamantane derivatives and used as the pretargeting vector. Poly(isobutyl methacrylate) (PIMBA) functionalized with 10 β-cyclodextrin handles was used as the pretargeting agent (**Table 4**) [62].

2.3.7 Comparison of the pretargeting strategies

Pretargeting system	*Rate constants [$M^{-1}\,s^{-1}$]*	*In vivo stability*	*Clinical studies*	*Benefits and limitations*
bsAb	$10^{3\text{–}5}$	High	Yes	+ Highly specific binding to variety of cellular targets + Straight forward accessibility through dock-and-lock approach - Reversible binding between hapten and bsAb - Lower tumor uptake compared to other methods
PNA	10^5	High	No	+ Stable to enzymatic degradation + Potentially allows for administering two different complementary strands - Increased complexity to incorporate clearing agents - Challenging preparation
SPAAC	10^{-1}–10^{-2}	Low	No	+ Easy access to pretargeting pairs - Low reactivity requires high molar ratios between pretargeting pairs
TCO-Tz ligation	$10^{3\text{–}6}$	Moderate	No	+ Excellent speed kinetics - Tetrazine synthesis challenging

Table 4.
Comparison of the pretargeting strategies utilized in pretargeted theranostics [4].

3. Conclusion

The recently seen rapid increase in development of novel pretargeted conjugation strategies allowed for pretargeted PET imaging and α/β^--therapy resulting in lower off-target toxicity and overall radiation doses. Despite preclinical successes, the increased complexity of the pretargeting approach still hampers further clinical translation, resulting in only few pretargeted theranostics being clinically investigated. Since the required multicomponent approach comes with high entry barriers of current good manufacturing practice (cGMP) production, the pretargeting approach must result in undoubtful benefits over more traditional imaging or treatment options. Although theranostics come with the large benefit of combining imaging and therapeutic agents, allowing for optimized treatment parameters, still more clinical trials need to be initiated and deliver prove of increased efficacy and decreased off-target toxicity to justify the inherently increased treatment challenges.

Acknowledgements

C.B.M.P acknowledges funding by the BRIDGE – Translational Excellence Programme at the Faculty of Health and Medical Sciences, University of Copenhagen, funded by the Novo Nordisk Foundation (grant agreement no.

NNF18SA0034956). Further, this project has received funding from the European Union's EU Framework Programme for Research and Innovation Horizon 2020, under grant agreement no. 668532.

Conflict of interest

The authors declare no competing financial interest.

Author details

Markus Staudt[1], Matthias M. Herth[1,2*] and Christian B.M. Poulie[1*]

1 Department of Drug Design and Pharmacology, University of Copenhagen, Copenhagen, Denmark

2 Department of Clinical Physiology, Nuclear Medicine and PET, Rigshospitalet, University Hospital, Copenhagen, Denmark

*Address all correspondence to: matthias.herth@sund.ku.dk and christian.poulie@sund.ku.dk

References

[1] S. Jeelani, R. Jagat Reddy, T. Maheswaran, G. Asokan, A. Dany, and B. Anand, "Theranostics: A treasured tailor for tomorrow," *J. Pharm. Bioallied Sci.*, vol. 6, no. 5, p. 6, 2014, doi: 10.4103/0975-7406.137249.

[2] S. Shrivastava, S. Jain, D. Kumar, S. L. Soni, and M. Sharma, "A Review on Theranostics: An Approach to Targeted Diagnosis and Therapy," *Asian J. Pharm. Res. Dev.*, vol. 7, no. 2, pp. 63-69, Apr. 2019, doi: 10.22270/ajprd.v7i2.463.

[3] E. J. L. Stéen *et al.*, "Pretargeting in nuclear imaging and radionuclide therapy: Improving efficacy of theranostics and nanomedicines," *Biomaterials*, vol. 179, pp. 209-245, Oct. 2018, doi: 10.1016/j.biomaterials.2018.06.021.

[4] E. J. L. Stéen *et al.*, "Pretargeting in nuclear imaging and radionuclide therapy: Improving efficacy of theranostics and nanomedicines," *Biomaterials*, vol. 179, pp. 209-245, Oct. 2018, doi: 10.1016/j.biomaterials.2018.06.021.

[5] S. Hapuarachchige and D. Artemov, "Theranostic Pretargeting Drug Delivery and Imaging Platforms in Cancer Precision Medicine," *Front. Oncol.*, vol. 10, Jul. 2020, doi: 10.3389/fonc.2020.01131.

[6] F. C. J. van de Watering, M. Rijpkema, M. Robillard, W. J. G. Oyen, and O. C. Boerman, "Pretargeted Imaging and Radioimmunotherapy of Cancer Using Antibodies and Bioorthogonal Chemistry," *Front. Med.*, vol. 1, Nov. 2014, doi: 10.3389/fmed.2014.00044.

[7] U. Eberlein, M. Cremonesi, and M. Lassmann, "Individualized Dosimetry for Theranostics: Necessary, Nice to Have, or Counterproductive?," *J. Nucl. Med.*, vol. 58, no. Supplement 2, pp. 97S–103S, Sep. 2017, doi: 10.2967/jnumed.116.186841.

[8] T. F. Massoud, "Molecular imaging in living subjects: seeing fundamental biological processes in a new light," *Genes Dev.*, vol. 17, no. 5, pp. 545-580, Mar. 2003, doi: 10.1101/gad.1047403.

[9] O. Arrieta, L.-A. Medina, E. Estrada-Lobato, L.-A. Ramírez-Tirado, V.-O. Mendoza-García, and J. de la Garza-Salazar, "High liposomal doxorubicin tumour tissue distribution, as determined by radiopharmaceutical labelling with 99mTc-LD, is associated with the response and survival of patients with unresectable pleural mesothelioma treated with a combination of liposomal doxorubicin and cisplatin," *Cancer Chemother. Pharmacol.*, vol. 74, no. 1, pp. 211-215, Jul. 2014, doi: 10.1007/s00280-014-2477-x.

[10] W. W. Moses, "Fundamental limits of spatial resolution in PET," *Nucl. Instruments Methods Phys. Res. Sect. A Accel. Spectrometers, Detect. Assoc. Equip.*, vol. 648, pp. S236–S240, Aug. 2011, doi: 10.1016/j.nima.2010.11.092.

[11] A. Rahmim and H. Zaidi, "PET versus SPECT: strengths, limitations and challenges," *Nucl. Med. Commun.*, vol. 29, no. 3, pp. 193-207, Mar. 2008, doi: 10.1097/MNM.0b013e3282f3a515.

[12] M. M. Herth, V. L. Andersen, S. Lehel, J. Madsen, G. M. Knudsen, and J. L. Kristensen, "Development of a 11C-labeled tetrazine for rapid tetrazine–trans-cyclooctene ligation," *Chem. Commun.*, vol. 49, no. 36, p. 3805, 2013, doi: 10.1039/c3cc41027g.

[13] S. M. Ametamey, M. Honer, and P. A. Schubiger, "Molecular Imaging with PET," *Chem. Rev.*, vol. 108, no. 5,

pp. 1501-1516, May 2008, doi: 10.1021/cr0782426.

[14] C. Ash, M. Dubec, K. Donne, and T. Bashford, “Effect of wavelength and beam width on penetration in light-tissue interaction using computational methods,” *Lasers Med. Sci.*, vol. 32, no. 8, pp. 1909-1918, Nov. 2017, doi: 10.1007/s10103-017-2317-4.

[15] R. E. Hendrick, “Spatial Resolution in Magnetic Resonance Imaging,” in *Breast MRI*, New York, NY: Springer New York, 2008, pp. 31-45.

[16] E. Blumfield, D. W. Swenson, R. S. Iyer, and A. L. Stanescu, “Gadolinium-based contrast agents — review of recent literature on magnetic resonance imaging signal intensity changes and tissue deposits, with emphasis on pediatric patients,” *Pediatr. Radiol.*, vol. 49, no. 4, pp. 448-457, Apr. 2019, doi: 10.1007/s00247-018-4304-8.

[17] R. A. Cloyd, S. A. Koren, and J. F. Abisambra, “Manganese-Enhanced Magnetic Resonance Imaging: Overview and Central Nervous System Applications With a Focus on Neurodegeneration,” *Front. Aging Neurosci.*, vol. 10, Dec. 2018, doi: 10.3389/fnagi.2018.00403.

[18] Y.-D. Xiao, R. Paudel, J. Liu, C. Ma, Z.-S. Zhang, and S.-K. Zhou, “MRI contrast agents: Classification and application (Review),” *Int. J. Mol. Med.*, vol. 38, no. 5, pp. 1319-1326, Nov. 2016, doi: 10.3892/ijmm.2016.2744.

[19] F. Zoller, M. Eisenhut, U. Haberkorn, and W. Mier, “Endoradiotherapy in cancer treatment — Basic concepts and future trends,” *Eur. J. Pharmacol.*, vol. 625, no. 1-3, pp. 55-62, Dec. 2009, doi: 10.1016/j.ejphar.2009.05.035.

[20] A. Morgenstern, F. Bruchertseifer, and C. Apostolidis, “Bismuth-213 and Actinium-225 – Generator Performance and Evolving Therapeutic Applications of Two Generator-Derived Alpha-Emitting Radioisotopes,” *Curr. Radiopharm.*, vol. 5, no. 3, pp. 221-227, Jun. 2012, doi: 10.2174/1874471011205030221.

[21] D. A. Scheinberg and M. R. McDevitt, “Actinium-225 in targeted alpha-particle therapeutic applications.,” *Curr. Radiopharm.*, vol. 4, no. 4, pp. 306-20, Oct. 2011, doi: 10.2174/1874471011104040306.

[22] S. Davies, B. J. Stenton, and G. J. L. Bernardes, “Bioorthogonal Decaging Reactions for Targeted Drug Activation,” *Chim. Int. J. Chem.*, vol. 72, no. 11, pp. 771-776, Nov. 2018, doi: 10.2533/chimia.2018.771.

[23] X. Ji *et al.*, “Click and release: bioorthogonal approaches to ‘on-demand’ activation of prodrugs,” *Chem. Soc. Rev.*, vol. 48, no. 4, pp. 1077-1094, 2019, doi: 10.1039/C8CS00395E.

[24] M. Czuban *et al.*, “Bio-Orthogonal Chemistry and Reloadable Biomaterial Enable Local Activation of Antibiotic Prodrugs and Enhance Treatments against *Staphylococcus aureus* Infections,” *ACS Cent. Sci.*, vol. 4, no. 12, pp. 1624-1632, Dec. 2018, doi: 10.1021/acscentsci.8b00344.

[25] R. Rossin *et al.*, “Chemically triggered drug release from an antibody-drug conjugate leads to potent antitumour activity in mice,” *Nat. Commun.*, vol. 9, no. 1, p. 1484, Dec. 2018, doi: 10.1038/s41467-018-03880-y.

[26] S. Hapuarachchige, Y. Kato, and D. Artemov, “Bioorthogonal two-component drug delivery in HER2(+) breast cancer mouse models,” *Sci. Rep.*, vol. 6, no. 1, p. 24298, Jul. 2016, doi: 10.1038/srep24298.

[27] G. R. Ediriweera *et al.*, “Targeted and modular architectural polymers employing bioorthogonal chemistry

for quantitative therapeutic delivery," *Chem. Sci.*, vol. 11, no. 12, pp. 3268-3280, 2020, doi: 10.1039/D0SC00078G.

[28] A. Forero *et al.*, "Phase 1 trial of a novel anti-CD20 fusion protein in pretargeted radioimmunotherapy for B-cell non-Hodgkin lymphoma," *Blood*, vol. 104, no. 1, pp. 227-236, Jul. 2004, doi: 10.1182/blood-2003-09-3284.

[29] G. Paganelli *et al.*, "Pre-targeted locoregional radioimmunotheraphy with 90Y-biotin in glioma patients: Phase I study and preliminary therapeutic results," *Cancer Biother. Radiopharm.*, vol. 16, no. 3, pp. 227-235, Jul. 2001, doi: 10.1089/10849780152389410.

[30] S. J. Knox *et al.*, "Phase II trial of yttrium-90-DOTA-biotin pretargeted by NR-LU-10 antibody/streptavidin in patients with metastatic colon cancer," *Clin. Cancer Res.*, vol. 6, no. 2, pp. 406-414, 2000.

[31] H. P. Kalofonos *et al.*, "Imaging of tumor in patients with indium-111-labeled biotin and streptavidin-conjugated antibodies: Preliminary communication," *J. Nucl. Med.*, 1990.

[32] H. B. Breitz *et al.*, "Clinical optimization of pretargeted radioimmunotherapy with antibody-streptavidin conjugate and 90Y-DOTA-biotin," *J. Nucl. Med.*, vol. 41, no. 1, pp. 131-140, 2000.

[33] A. Bates and C. A. Power, "David vs. Goliath: The Structure, Function, and Clinical Prospects of Antibody Fragments," *Antibodies*, 2019, doi: 10.3390/antib8020028.

[34] S. M. Cheal *et al.*, "Curative multicycle radioimmunotherapy monitored by quantitative SPECT/CT-based theranostics, using bispecific antibody pretargeting strategy in colorectal cancer," *J. Nucl. Med.*, vol. 58, no. 11, pp. 1735-1742, Nov. 2017, doi: 10.2967/jnumed.117.193250.

[35] S. M. Cheal *et al.*, "Theranostic pretargeted radioimmunotherapy of internalizing solid tumor antigens in human tumor xenografts in mice: Curative treatment of HER2-positive breast carcinoma," *Theranostics*, vol. 8, no. 18, pp. 5106-5125, 2018, doi: 10.7150/thno.26585.

[36] K. D. Orcutt *et al.*, "Engineering an antibody with picomolar affinity to DOTA chelates of multiple radionuclides for pretargeted radioimmunotherapy and imaging," *Nucl. Med. Biol.*, vol. 38, no. 2, pp. 223-233, 2011, doi: 10.1016/j.nucmedbio.2010.08.013.

[37] S. M. Cheal *et al.*, "Theranostic pretargeted radioimmunotherapy of colorectal cancer xenografts in mice using picomolar affinity 86Y- or 177Lu-DOTA-Bn binding scFv C825/GPA33 IgG bispecific immunoconjugates," *Eur. J. Nucl. Med. Mol. Imaging*, vol. 43, no. 5, pp. 925-937, May 2016, doi: 10.1007/s00259-015-3254-8.

[38] S. M. Cheal *et al.*, "Alpha radioimmunotherapy using 225Ac-proteus-DOTA for solid tumors – Safety at curative doses," *Theranostics*, vol. 10, no. 25, pp. 11359-11375, 2020, doi: 10.7150/thno.48810.

[39] F. C. J. van de Watering, M. Rijpkema, M. Robillard, W. J. G. Oyen, and O. C. Boerman, "Pretargeted Imaging and Radioimmunotherapy of Cancer Using Antibodies and Bioorthogonal Chemistry," *Front. Med.*, vol. 1, Nov. 2014, doi: 10.3389/fmed.2014.00044.

[40] R. Schoffelen *et al.*, "Pretargeted immuno-positron emission tomography imaging of carcinoembryonic antigen-expressing tumors with a bispecific antibody and a68Ga- And18F-labeled hapten peptide in mice with human

tumor xenografts," *Mol. Cancer Ther.*, vol. 9, no. 4, pp. 1019-1027, Apr. 2010, doi: 10.1158/1535-7163.MCT-09-0862.

[41] R. Schoffelen *et al.*, "Quantitative immuno-SPECT monitoring of pretargeted radioimmunotherapy with a bispecific antibody in an intraperitoneal nude mouse model of human colon cancer," *J. Nucl. Med.*, vol. 53, no. 12, pp. 1926-1932, 2012, doi: 10.2967/jnumed.112.106278.

[42] S. Heskamp *et al.*, "α-Versus β-Emitting radionuclides for pretargeted radioimmunotherapy of carcinoembryonic antigen-expressing human colon cancer xenografts," *J. Nucl. Med.*, vol. 58, no. 6, pp. 926-933, Jun. 2017, doi: 10.2967/jnumed.116.187021.

[43] R. Schoffelen *et al.*, "Development of an imaging-guided CEA-pretargeted radionuclide treatment of advanced colorectal cancer: First clinical results," *Br. J. Cancer*, vol. 109, no. 4, pp. 934-942, 2013, doi: 10.1038/bjc.2013.376.

[44] C. Bodet-Milin *et al.*, "Pharmacokinetics and dosimetry studies for optimization of pretargeted radioimmunotherapy in CEA-expressing advanced lung cancer patients," *Front. Med.*, vol. 2, no. NOV, p. 27, Nov. 2015, doi: 10.3389/fmed.2015.00084.

[45] V. V. Demidov *et al.*, "Stability of peptide nucleic acids in human serum and cellular extracts," *Biochem. Pharmacol.*, 1994, doi: 10.1016/0006-2952(94)90171-6.

[46] D. S. Youngblood, S. A. Hatlevig, J. N. Hassinger, P. L. Iversen, and H. M. Moulton, "Stability of cell-penetrating peptide-morpholino oligomer conjugates in human serum and in cells," *Bioconjug. Chem.*, vol. 18, no. 1, pp. 50-60, Jan. 2007, doi: 10.1021/bc060138s.

[47] A. Vorobyeva *et al.*, "Development of an optimal imaging strategy for selection of patients for affibody-based PNA-mediated radionuclide therapy," *Sci. Rep.*, vol. 8, no. 1, p. 9643, Dec. 2018, doi: 10.1038/s41598-018-27886-0.

[48] A. Vorobyeva *et al.*, "Development of an optimal imaging strategy for selection of patients for affibody-based PNA-mediated radionuclide therapy," *Sci. Rep.*, vol. 8, no. 1, p. 9643, Dec. 2018, doi: 10.1038/s41598-018-27886-0.

[49] B. L. Oliveira, Z. Guo, and G. J. L. Bernardes, "Inverse electron demand Diels–Alder reactions in chemical biology," *Chem. Soc. Rev.*, vol. 46, no. 16, pp. 4895-4950, 2017, doi: 10.1039/C7CS00184C.

[50] P. E. Edem *et al.*, "Evaluation of the inverse electron demand Diels-Alder reaction in rats using a scandium-44-labelled tetrazine for pretargeted PET imaging," *EJNMMI Res.*, vol. 9, no. 1, p. 49, Dec. 2019, doi: 10.1186/s13550-019-0520-y.

[51] E. J. L. Stéen *et al.*, "Trans -Cyclooctene-Functionalized PeptoBrushes with Improved Reaction Kinetics of the Tetrazine Ligation for Pretargeted Nuclear Imaging," *ACS Nano*, vol. 14, no. 1, pp. 568-584, Jan. 2020, doi: 10.1021/acsnano.9b06905.

[52] A. Rondon *et al.*, "Pretargeted radioimmunotherapy and SPECT imaging of peritoneal carcinomatosis using bioorthogonal click chemistry: probe selection and first proof-of-concept," *Theranostics*, vol. 9, no. 22, pp. 6706-6718, 2019, doi: 10.7150/thno.35461.

[53] O. Keinänen *et al.*, "Dual Radionuclide Theranostic Pretargeting," *Mol. Pharm.*, vol. 16, no. 10, pp. 4416-4421, 2019, doi: 10.1021/acs.molpharmaceut.9b00746.

[54] O. Keinänen *et al.*, "Harnessing 64 Cu/67 Cu for a theranostic approach to

pretargeted radioimmunotherapy," *Proc. Natl. Acad. Sci.*, p. 202009960, Oct. 2020, doi: 10.1073/pnas.2009960117.

[55] S. Hapuarachchige, Y. Kato, and D. Artemov, "Bioorthogonal two-component drug delivery in HER2(+) breast cancer mouse models," *Sci. Rep.*, vol. 6, no. 1, p. 24298, Jul. 2016, doi: 10.1038/srep24298.

[56] S. Hapuarachchige *et al.*, "Cellular Delivery of Bioorthogonal Pretargeting Therapeutics in PSMA-Positive Prostate Cancer," *Mol. Pharm.*, vol. 17, no. 1, pp. 98-108, Jan. 2020, doi: 10.1021/acs.molpharmaceut.9b00788.

[57] R. Rossin *et al.*, "Chemically triggered drug release from an antibody-drug conjugate leads to potent antitumour activity in mice," *Nat. Commun.*, vol. 9, no. 1, p. 1484, Dec. 2018, doi: 10.1038/s41467-018-03880-y.

[58] G. R. Ediriweera *et al.*, "Targeted and modular architectural polymers employing bioorthogonal chemistry for quantitative therapeutic delivery," *Chem. Sci.*, vol. 11, no. 12, pp. 3268-3280, 2020, doi: 10.1039/D0SC00078G.

[59] I. Khan, P. F. Agris, M. V. Yigit, and M. Royzen, "In situ activation of a doxorubicin prodrug using imaging-capable nanoparticles," *Chem. Commun.*, vol. 52, no. 36, pp. 6174-6177, 2016, doi: 10.1039/C6CC01024E.

[60] B. L. Oliveira, Z. Guo, and G. J. L. Bernardes, "Inverse electron demand Diels–Alder reactions in chemical biology," *Chem. Soc. Rev.*, vol. 46, no. 16, pp. 4895-4950, 2017, doi: 10.1039/C7CS00184C.

[61] M. R. Eftink, M. L. Andy, K. Bystrom, H. D. Perlmutter, and D. S. Kristol, "Cyclodextrin inclusion complexes: studies of the variation in the size of alicyclic guests," *J. Am. Chem. Soc.*, vol. 111, no. 17, pp. 6765-6772, Aug. 1989, doi: 10.1021/ja00199a041.

[62] S. J. Spa *et al.*, "A Supramolecular Approach for Liver Radioembolization," *Theranostics*, vol. 8, no. 9, pp. 2377-2386, 2018, doi: 10.7150/thno.23567.

Section 2

Theranostics Based on Naturally Occuring Components

Chapter 3

Aptamers: Magic Bullet for Theranostic Applications

Arghya Sett

Abstract

Aptamers are a short polymer of oligonucleotides (natural or modified) that can bind to its cognate target (small molecules to large macromolecules like proteins, cells, microorganisms etc.) with high affinity and selectivity. They can fold into unique secondary and tertiary conformation in solution (pH, ionic concentration) and bind to their targets in a specific manner (binding constants in sub-nano to pico molar range). They rival the monoclonal antibodies and other specific biological ligands with respect to affinity, stability, robustness, non-immunogenicity and facile to synthesis. Nucleic acid aptamers are selected from an oligonucleotide library by an iterative process called SELEX (**S**ystematic **E**volution of **L**igands by **Ex**ponential Enrichment Analysis). These aptamers are compatible to any kind of chemical modification, conjugation and functionalization. Briefly, this chapter discusses about the diagnostic and therapeutic application of aptamers.

Keywords: aptamers, SELEX, theranostics, chemical antibodies

1. Introduction

Aptamers (Latin word *aptus* means 'to fit' and Greek meros meaning 'part') are single stranded oligonucleotides, which act as synthetic ligands for its cognate target molecules. [1, 2] These molecules show high target specificity, selectivity and affinity, which resemble 'monoclonal antibody'. Similar to antibodies, aptamers also have immense potential to interact with their targets by structural recognition and thus they are termed as 'chemical antibodies'. [3] Different conformations allow aptamers to bind specifically with their target by 'lock and key' model. This hypothesis of binding mechanism is driven by the secondary and tertiary structure of aptamers in-bound state with their targets. Adopting various structures like hairpin loops, bulges, stem-loop, quartets, G-quadruplex, pseudo knots, aptamers can fit into the binding region of the target. [4] Intra and inter molecular interactions like hydrogen bonding, Vander Waals force, hydrophobic interaction, electrostatic forces play major crucial role in aptamer-target interaction. [5] However, the aptamers are primarily synthetic molecules and naturally occurring ribozymes are single stranded RNA molecules, which also have similar recognition domain acting in a similar manner. [6, 7] Aptamers are capable of forming various stable three-dimensional structures in physiological solution. The folding process in solution and the ligand-induced conformational switch is strongly dependent on the presence of divalent cations (magnesium, potassium etc.). [8] There are plethora of computer algorithms enable sequence based modeling of secondary structure of the oligonucleotide aptamers which actually strengthen the predictability of strongest binders with lowest free energy. [9, 10] Aptamers fold into tertiary conformations and bind to their targets through shape complementarity at the aptamer-target interface. [11] An aptamer binds to a protein can modulate protein functions by interfering with protein interaction with natural partners. Similar to antibodies, aptamers can enter to specific target cells via receptor-mediated endocytosis upon binding to cell surface ligands. [12] Importantly, aptamers can penetrate into tumor cores much more efficiently than antibodies due to their ~20–25-fold smaller sizes compared with full sized monoclonal antibodies. [13, 14]

Monoclonal Antibody	Aptamer
Stability: Monoclonal antibodies require refrigeration to avoid denaturation. Limited shelf life. [15]	**Stability:** Aptamers do not require refrigeration. Indefinite shelf life. [16]
Immunogenicity: They can cause immunogenic response. [17]	**Immunogenicity:** Aptamers are non-immunogenic. [18]
Production: laborious, expensive, high batch-to-batch variation.	**Production:** simpler and controlled chemical reactions, little to no variation, automated, chemical synthesis, no contamination.
Size: Larger in size, they can resist filtration by the kidneys, long half-lives. However, their size prevents access to smaller areas. [19]	**Size:** Aptamers are small molecules. They are especially subject to kidney filtration, resulting in short half-lives. Compared to antibodies, aptamers can bind to smaller targets. [20]
Ability to modification: Antibodies cannot accommodate conjugates without negative consequences such as reduced activity.	**Ability to modification:** Easy to modify, modifications can also be incorporated during synthesis to prevent kidney filtration. [21]

Table 1.
Comparison between Monoclonal antibody vs. Aptamer:

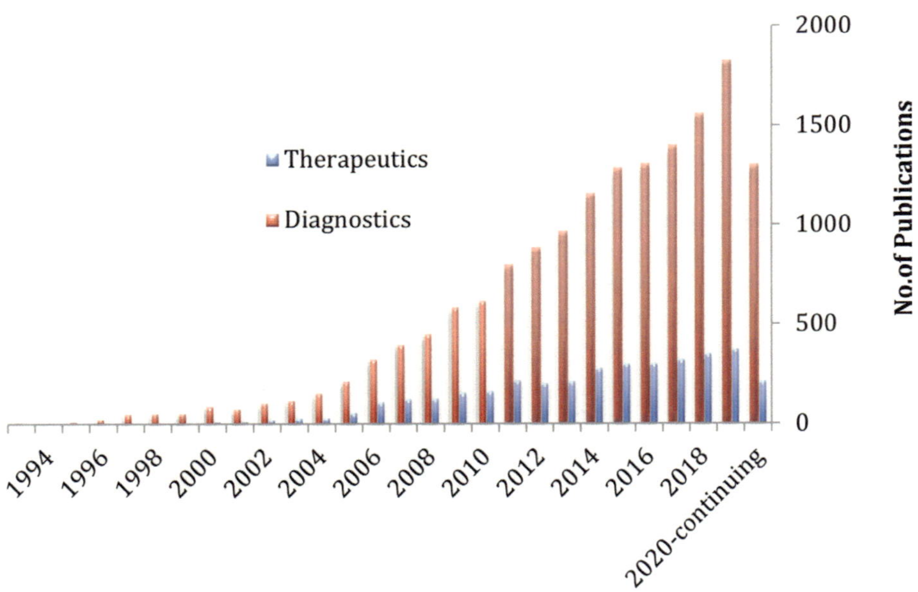

Figure 1.
Publication trend for Search strings: "Aptamers as diagnostics" and "Aptamers as therapeutics" (Source: Scopus).

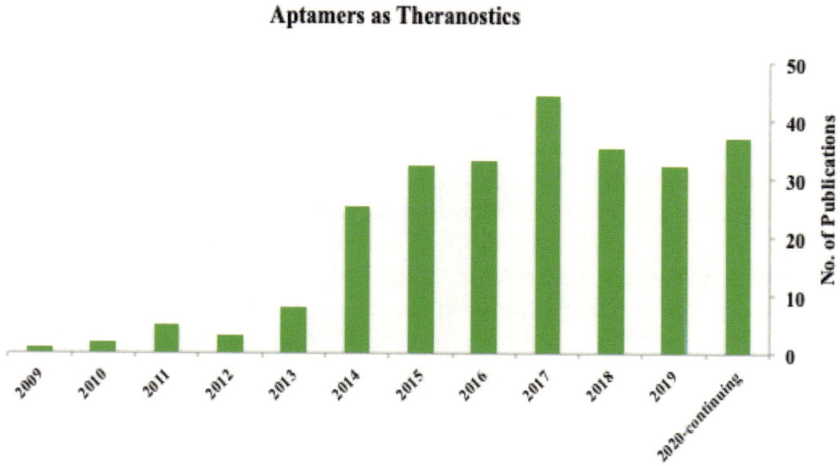

Figure 2.
Publication trend for Search strings: "Aptamers as theranostics" (Source: Scopus).

Compared to antibodies, aptamers can be produced using cell-free chemical synthesis and are therefore less expensive for large-scale manufacture. Aptamers exhibit extremely low variability between batches and have better controlled post-production modification, they are minimally immunogenic, and are small in size. (**Table 1**) The rapidly growing aptamer industry was predicted to reach US $244.93 million by 2020. [22] Presently more than 40 companies are actively engaged in diagnostics and therapeutics research to commercialize these "magic bullets" globally (EU countries, Asia, USA, UK etc.). [23] The largest company is "SomaLogic" (company based on SOMAmer- a patented "Slow Off-rate Modified Aptamer) founded by Prof. Larry Gold at Colorado, USA. Since the advent of aptamers scientists and researchers exploit different applications of aptamers that reflects the following trends in the publications. (**Figures 1** and **2**).

2. Basics of SELEX screening process

Back in 1990, two individual groups Prof. Larry Gold and Craig Tuerk from University of Boulder, USA and Prof. Jack Szostak and his student A.D. Ellington from Havard University, USA discovered the evolution process to obtain the oligonucleotide binders and they coined the term 'Aptamer' and the process as 'SELEX'. [24, 25] Systematic Evolution of Ligands by Exponential Enrichment (SELEX) is a common screening process by which aptamers can be selected from an aptamer library which consist of 10^{24-25} number of various sequences. The method attempts to isolate an aptamer of interest from a pool of randomized library by an iterative cycle of incubation with the target, partitioning and amplification, until the pool of aptamers enriched enough to fit with the target. The SELEX procedure iterates over five basic steps- incubation of aptamer pools with the target, binding, partitioning and washing (to get rid of non-binders which are loosely bound with the target), then elution of positive target-bound aptamers and amplification of enriched pools. Traditionally, the positive pool eluted from last round is being analysed, and high-throughput sequencing is performed.

An array of different RNA and DNA aptamers were isolated against a vast array of targets: ions, [26] low molecular weight metabolites, [27, 28] proteins, [29–31] sugar moieties [32] lipids, [33] and even whole cells. [34, 35]

3. Library selection

To select highly selective, specific aptamers, design of the initial aptamer library is the first and foremost step. In case of determination of the length of the random region researchers should consider the sequence space and structural diversity. The complexity of the initial aptamer library depends on the length of the random window of the aptamer library (If the random window is 40 and if we consider DNA aptamer library, so the complexity of the library is: 4^40 that equals to 10^{24-25}). [36]

Special libraries would consist of specifically designed flanking sequences directing the aptamers to form a specific secondary structure, or include modified nucleotides. In capture SELEX, there is unique docking sequence (12–14 nucleotides long) which enables the library in such a way, that highly sensitive aptamers can be fished out against small molecules. [37, 38] The extended genetic alphabets or combination of artificial xeno nucleic acids (XNA) greatly broaden the diversity of sequences and can influence the properties of the aptamers, such as their in vivo stability or nuclease resistance. [39–42] Modified nucleotides can be introduced either during the library synthesis or in the post-selection optimization.

In a review article, Maria *et al.* summarized all key features of designing nucleic acid libraries for SELEX like nature, composition of the library (RNA, DNA or modified nucleotides), the length of a randomized region and the presence of fixed sequences. Different randomization strategies and computer algorithms of library designs were also discussed. [43]

4. Various SELEX processes

Specific aptamers are screened by the iterative processs of SELEX from a highly diverse pool of oligonucleotides. [44–46] After the incubation of the random aptamer pool with the target followed by the removal of non- binding aptamers, the bound aptamer species are recovered. These recovered nucleic acid sequences are amplified with PCR (in the case of DNA aptamer) or RT-PCR (for RNA aptamers). In addition to selection against a purified target molecule, SELEX process can be performed against live bacterial cells and even in mammalian cell lines to isolate cancer cell specific aptamers and furthermore it can lead to the identification of novel biomarkers. [47, 48]

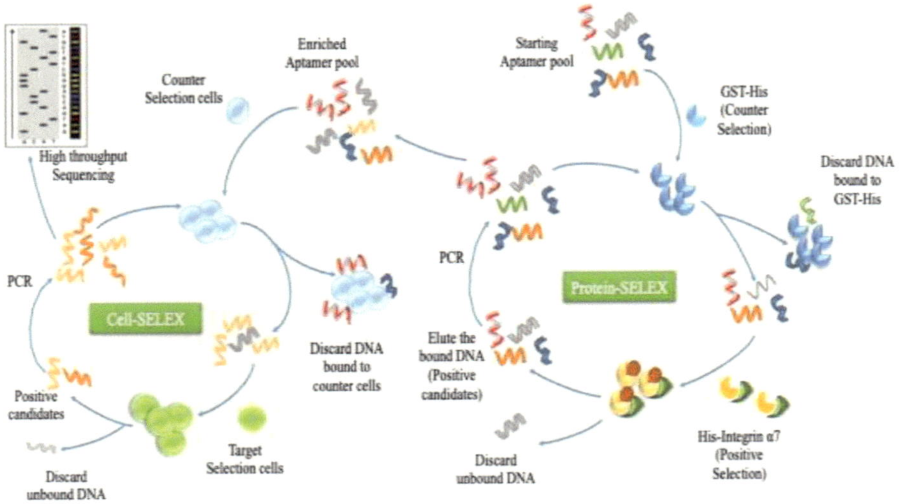

Figure 3.
Typical schema of Cross-over SELEX process.

A giant advancement of SELEX technology has been made since its discovery in 1990. Conventional SELEX is a well-established and effective method but due to its immense time- and labor-consumption, continuous improvement of alternative methods for aptamer selection has been inevitable.

High throughput SELEX (HT-SELEX), Functional screening (Microfludics or Flow cytometry based SELEX), Cross-over SELEX (where the target is alternatively changing from proteins and cells), (**Figure 3**) *in-vivo* SELEX, Spiegelmers selection, de-convolution SELEX are few examples of modern-era screening strategy of aptamers. [49] Cutting-edge functional screening process, the chemical modifications, Next-generation sequencing (NGS technology) enable SELEX more efficient, cost-effective and considerably less time-consuming.

5. Modifications of naturally occuring aptamers

DNA is the backbone of central dogma of our life cycle. Moreover, any form of nucleic acids play a crucial role in our genetic codon. DNA/RNA is an essential bio-macromolecule consist of nucleotide bases such as adenine (A), thymine (T), uracil (U), guanine (G), cytosine (C).

There are various types of modifications (nucleotide base modifications, phosphate backbone modifications, peptide mimic oligonucleotides PNA etc.) available which can prevent aptamers from nuclease degradation. Locked nucleic acid (LNA) is one among them where 2′-oxygen has been linked to the 4′-carbon of the ribose sugar by a methylene bridge, thus completely locking the sugar into a 3′-endo conformation. LNAs increase the thermodynamic stability, binding affinity, and enable the oligonucleotides to prevent serum degradation. [50–52] These modifications enable the aptamers for biological applications.

Compared to LNAs, the unlocked nucleic acid (UNA) is an acyclic ribose derivative that has increased flexibility. UNAs do not consist the C2'-C3' bond, which confers the flexibility observed in this modified nucleotide. [53] LNAs increase the melting temperature of the nucleotide by 1–10°C per LNA insertion but UNAs reduce the melting temperature by 5–10°C retaining the nuclear resistance. In case of, Peptide nucleic acid (PNA) in which sugar-phosphate backbone is modified by short stretch of N-(2-aminoethyl)-glycine units connected by peptide bonds, enhances biostability of the modified candidates. [54]

5.1 Aptamers in Drug development pipeline

Aptamers have been incorporated in drug development pipeline as they have the capacity to block the downstream signalling (phosphorylation of kinases etc.) of different biomolecules. They can play an important role to regulate various cellular crosstalks. To screen therapeutic aptamers either DNA aptamers or 2′-fluoro modified RNA, a combination of 2′-fluoro pyrimidines and 2′-hydroxyl purines (fYrR) are of major interest. fYrR is the "nuclease stable RNA" and can be easily generated by Y639F modified T7 RNA polymerase. Fovista, an anti-platelet derived growth factor (PDGF) aptamer, was previously DNA aptamer but later modified to augment the stability with the addition of backbone modifications. [55] As with the 2′-fluoro modification, the 2'-OMe modifications adopt a C3'-endo conformation. US FDA approved the first aptamer (Macugen®, pegaptanib sodium) in 2004 against vascular endothelial growth factor for the treatment of age-related macular degeneration. [56] This aptamer was modified with 2′-fluoro-pyrimidines and 2'-O-methyl-purines. The stability of the small aptamer was a critical factor but later which can be circumvented with a 3′-cap and a polyethylene glycol molecule, the half-life of Macugen® was extended to 131 hours at max. [57, 58] Anti-vascular endothelial growth factor (VEGF 165) aptamer Macugen, and an anti-Factor IXa aptamer REG1 were both selected from fYrR libraries, and subsequently 2′-O-methyl nucleosides have been incorporated in order to increase serum stability. [57]

There is a plethora of polymerase enzymes like KOD, Pwo, Phusion, Superscript III, vent (exo-), T7 polymerase have all been shown to be capable of incorporating modified triphosphates into DNA and RNA strands, which open up a new opportunities in aptamer selection strategies. [59] The use of Pfx DNA polymerase allows amplification of Ds-Px base pair in Ex-SELEX protocol where extended genetic alphabets were included in complexity of nucleic acid library. [60]

Several limitations of aptamers should be considered in the process of *in-vivo* applications of nucleic acid aptamers. Being polynucleotides, nucleic acid aptamers are naturally susceptible to enzymes degradation by exo and/or endo-nucleases, leading to a reduced *in vivo* circulatory half-life. This drawback can be alleviated by side chain chemical modifications to aptamers, incorporating unnatural nucleotide bases (locked and unlocked nucleic acids) and capping the aptamer ends, thus minimizing the susceptibility to endonuclease and exonuclease attack. [50, 51] Short blood residence time is another challenge with in vivo aptamer applications, which is due to fast removal of aptamer from the circulation by renal filtration as most aptamers have a size smaller than the renal filtration threshold of 40 kDa. [31] To achieve desired serum half-life, aptamers can be engineered by conjugation with a terminal polyethylene glycol (PEG), although this may compromise the extent of tumor penetration [61]. In some cases, post-SELEX modifications following the selection of aptamers may alter the 3-D structure of the aptamers, leading to the lost or altered binding affinity and specificity. Such problems can be prevented by using random aptamer pools containing modified nucleotides during the SELEX process. [62, 63] In addition, the ability of aptamers to interact with cells may decrease due to repulsion of nucleic acids by negatively-charged cell membranes. This can be refuted by increasing the binding affinity and specificity of aptamers toward their cell surface receptors to trigger receptor-mediated endocytosis.

In the field of oncology, two aptamers, namely, AS1411 and NOX-A12, have entered clinical trials. [45, 64] AS1411 (formerly ARGO100; Antisoma) is a guanine quadruplex aptamer obtained from a guanine-rich oligonucleotide library in the anti-proliferation screen, which is not a typical SELEX process. [65] The guanine quadruplex structure benefits AS1411 because it is resistant to nuclease degradation and enhances cell uptake. In *in-vitro* validations, AS1411 inhibits more than 80 types of cancer cell lines. In addition, the target of AS1411 has been verified to be nucleolin, and the relevant mechanism and specificity against cancer cells have also been described. In preclinical tests, AS1411 shows efficacy toward xenograft models, including non-small cell lung, renal, and breast cancers. It entered clinical trials in 2003 and passed phase II trials for acute myeloid leukemia. A subsequent phase II trial for renal cell carcinoma started in 2008 (clinical trial ID NCT00740441). [66] NOXA12 (Olaptesed pegol; Noxxon) is an L-form RNA aptamer known as Spiegelmer and is used for cancer therapy. NOX-A12 can bind to its target chemokine CXCL-12 and blocks its interaction with its receptor. [67] This disrupts the tissue gradient of CXCL-12 and reduces the cancer cell homing that might lead to tumor metastasis and drug resistance. [68] Currently, phase II clinical trials for NOX-A12 are underway for the treatment of chronic lymphocytic leukemia and refractory multiple myeloma (clinical trial IDs NCT01486797 and NCT01521533). [67] Aptamer based cancer therapeutics have immense potential for precise and less toxic treatment for cancer patients. [46]

6. Aptamers as diagnostic agents

Aptamers can be used *in-vitro* and *in-vivo* as well. [69] In terms of *in vivo* diagnostics, 'escort' aptamers can be implied as vehicles for a detectable molecules, such as radionuclides, fluorophores etc. [70–72] The development of new agents like radio-pharmaceuticals is challenging. There are some important factors such as efficiency of the radiolabeling process, specific activity (radioactivity per moles e.g. Ci/μmol), chemical purity, radiochemical and chemical stability and shelf life of the final product. [73] Mostly, radiolabeling strategies for aptamers are similar as for proteins, or antibodies. Aptamers can be easily chemically modified at its 5′ or 3′ end with a desired functional group for radiolabeling (**Figure 4**).

Radiohalogens (fluorine-18, bromine-76, iodine-125 etc.) are the most commonly used for radiolabelling oloigonuclotides which are often accompanied with prosthetic groups. Recently, click-chemistry for radiofluorination was demonstrated on antisense oligonucleotides and siRNAs. [74, 75] Another report used photoconjugation as strategy for the radiofluorination of an aptamer. [76] Oligonucleotides have also been radiolabeled with the radiohalogens such as bromine-76 for PET imaging and iodine-123 for SPECT (Single photon emission computed tomography) imaging. In addition, iodine-125 has been used to radiolabel antisense oligonucleotides, aptamers and spiegelmers for theranostic applications. Due to the harsh and non-aqueous reaction conditions usually needed to radiolabel prosthetic groups, it is performed before the conjugation process to the oligonucleotide. [73]

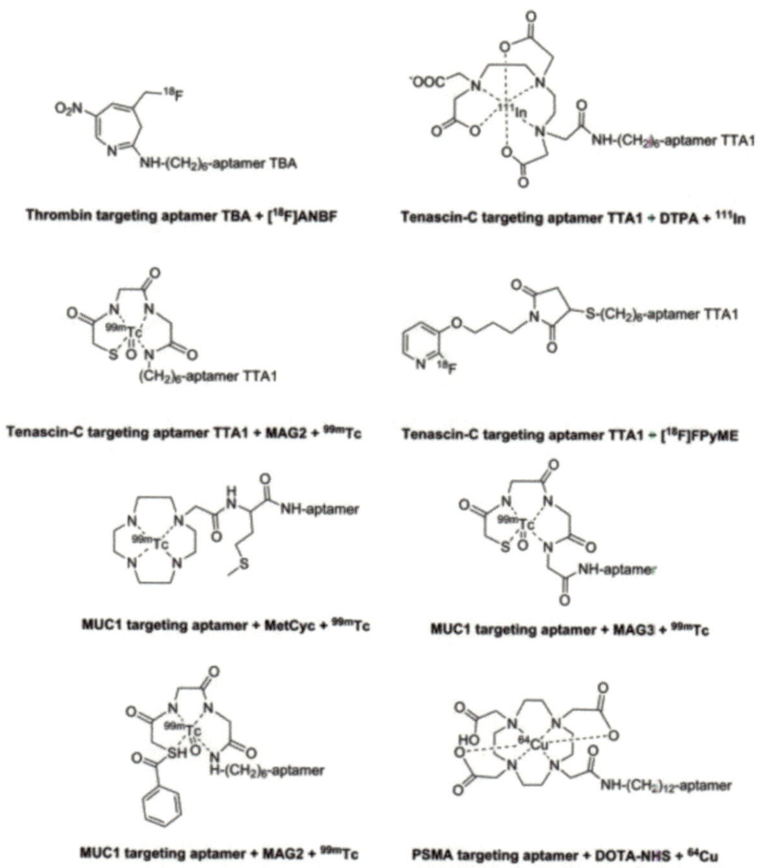

Figure 4.
Aptamers modified with radiolabelled molecules for disase diagnosis (Figure adapted from Gijs et al*) [73].*

Till date, a plethora of aptamers have been modified or labelled with radioactive molecules. Aptamers against several important biomarkers like PMSA, Tenascin C, thrombin, MUC1 were already exploited for radiolabelling. Aptamer-based radiopharmaceuticals were primarily developed for imaging and therapy of cancer diseases, metabolic disorders and others. The aptamers are mainly radiolabeled with technetium-99 m for SPECT (Single photon emission computed tomography), PET (Positron emission tomography) imaging. Very few aptamers were published related to PET imaging, and there is only one study of radiolabeled aptamers for therapy by Bandekar *et al.* [77] Other radiolabeled aptamers have only been tested for preclinical applications or in the course of preclinical assesement.

Molecular nuclear imaging technique is a diagnostic process of non-invasive visualization of any disease *in-vivo* at molecular level with high precision. For nuclear imaging, the probes used for radiolabelling has to be modified accordingly. Aptamers are the most promising candidates with versatile modification capibility, can be easily engineered for various imaging and other diagnostic purposes.

The first radiolabeled aptamer for nuclear imaging was discovered by Charlton et al. A DNA aptamer, NX21909, was selected against human neutrophil elastase, an enzyme which is secreted by neutrophils and macrophages during inflammation to kill pathogens. [78]

Aptamer TTA1, an RNA aptamer targeting the extracellular matrix protein tenascin C (TN-C), was the first radiolabeled aptamer which was used as molecular cancer imaging agent. Aptamer TTA1 was generated by a cross-over SELEX involving the purified recombinant TN-C protein and TN-C-positive U251 glioblastoma cells. [79, 80]

7. Lightup aptasensors for diagnostic applications

There are a unique group of aptamers (generally RNA aptamers) which can bind specifically with their cognate fluorogen molecules like DFHBI, thiazole orange, thioflavin T etc. [49, 81, 82] The non-fluorescent moelcules (native unbound state) become fluorescent (bound state) after binding to the aptamers and these "light-up" aptamers generate fluorescence signal. In the omni-presence of target molecules (small pre-miRNAs) and malachite green (fluorogen) light up aptasensors 'malaswitch' exhibit fluorescence enhancement. [83] We can engineer the small-molecule specific aptamers (like aptamers for some pesticides, toxins, small metaboltes) in such a way, that combined with light-up aptamers, they can generate a detectable signal. Light up aptasensors are promising alternative biosensor for label free sensitive detection of small molecules. [84]

8. Future perspectives

With more focus on *in vivo* studies for potential clinical applications, aptamers can be developed in combination with DNA nanostructures, nanomaterial, or microfluidic devices as diagnostic probes or therapeutic agents for cancers, infectious diseases, genetic, metabolic, neurological disorders, lifestyle diseases and several others. The use of aptamers as targeting agents in drug delivery can also be explored. Aptamers might be exploited to develop portable, low-cost and robust diagnostic kit using simple devices for real-time and on-site POC (point-of-care) detection and monitoring, instead of the laborious and time-consuming diagnostic tests currently available only in clinical labs. Regarding therapeutics approach, there is still untapped potential in the combination of the target recognition and strong binding property of aptamers with exquisitely designed nanomaterials. It can be used as an effective alternative drug delivery platform. Variety of materials such as liposomes, polymer vesicles and silica nanoparticles, combined with DNA/RNA aptamers, has shown feasibility for use in *in vivo* targeted drug delivery. [85, 86] The integration of diagnostic capability with therapeutic interventions termed, as "Theranostics" is critical to address the challenges of disease heterogeneity and adaptation. Although aptamers have immense potential as theranostic agents, tailor-made modifications, validation of experiments need to be executed before aptamer-based drug delivery can reach clinical trials and eventually the patient management system.

Author details

Arghya Sett
Institute of Organic Chemistry and Biochemistry, Academy of Sciences of the Czech Republic, Prague, Czech Republic

*Address all correspondence to: arghya.sett@gmail.com

References

[1] Famulok M, Mayer G. Aptamers and SELEX in chemistry & biology. Vol. 21, Chemistry and Biology. 2014.

[2] Nimjee SM, White RR, Becker RC, Sullenger BA. Aptamers as Therapeutics. Annu Rev Pharmacol Toxicol [Internet]. 2017 Jan 6;57:61-79. Available from: https://pubmed.ncbi.nlm.nih.gov/28061688

[3] Bauer M, Strom M, Hammond DS, Shigdar S. Anything You Can Do, I Can Do Better: Can Aptamers Replace Antibodies in Clinical Diagnostic Applications? Molecules. 2019;24(23):4377.

[4] Cai S, Yan J, Xiong H, Liu Y, Peng D, Liu Z. Investigations on the interface of nucleic acid aptamers and binding targets. Analyst [Internet]. 2018;143(22):5317-38. Available from: http://dx.doi.org/10.1039/C8AN01467A

[5] Elskens JP, Elskens JM, Madder A. Chemical Modification of Aptamers for Increased Binding Affinity in Diagnostic Applications: Current Status and Future Prospects. Int J Mol Sci. 2020;21(12):4522.

[6] Breaker RR, Joyce GF. The Expanding View of RNA and DNA Function. Chem Biol [Internet]. 2014;21(9):1059-65. Available from: http://linkinghub.elsevier.com/retrieve/pii/S1074552114002373

[7] Doudna JA, Cech TR. The chemical repertoire of natural ribozymes. Nature. 2002;418(6894):222-8.

[8] Horiya S, Li X, Kawai G, Saito R, Katoh A, Kobayashi K, et al. RNA LEGO: magnesium-dependent formation of specific RNA assemblies through kissing interactions. Chem Biol. 2003;10(7):645-54.

[9] Zuker M. Mfold web server for nucleic acid folding and hybridization prediction. Nucleic Acids Res [Internet]. 2003 Jul 1;31(13):3406-15. Available from: http://www.ncbi.nlm.nih.gov/pmc/articles/PMC169194/

[10] Wolfe BR, Porubsky NJ, Zadeh JN, Dirks RM, Pierce NA. Constrained multistate sequence design for nucleic acid reaction pathway engineering. J Am Chem Soc. 2017;139(8):3134-44.

[11] Khati M. The Future of Aptamers in Medicine. J Clin Pathol [Internet]. 2010;63(6):480-7. Available from: http://www.ncbi.nlm.nih.gov/pubmed/20360137

[12] Cibiel A, Dupont DM, Ducongé F. Methods to identify aptamers against cell surface biomarkers. Pharmaceuticals. 2011;4(9):1216-35.

[13] Soper SA, Brown K, Ellington A, Frazier B, Garcia-Manero G, Gau V, et al. Point-of-care biosensor systems for cancer diagnostics/prognostics. Biosens Bioelectron. 2006;21(10):1932-42.

[14] Brody EN, Willis MC, Smith JD, Jayasena S, Zichi D, Gold L. The use of aptamers in large arrays for molecular diagnostics. Vol. 4, Molecular Diagnosis. 1999. p. 381-8.

[15] Le Basle Y, Chennell P, Tokhadze N, Astier A, Sautou V. Physicochemical stability of monoclonal antibodies: a review. J Pharm Sci. 2020;109(1):169-90.

[16] Bruno JG. Long shelf life of a lyophilized DNA aptamer beacon assay. J Fluoresc. 2017;27(2):439-41.

[17] Kozlowski S, Swann P. Current and future issues in the manufacturing and development of monoclonal antibodies. Adv Drug Deliv Rev. 2006;58(5-6):707-22.

[18] Esposito CL, Passaro D, Longobardo I, Condorelli G, Marotta P, Affuso A, et al. A Neutralizing RNA Aptamer against EGFR Causes Selective Apoptotic Cell Death. PLoS One [Internet]. 2011;6(9):e24071. Available from: http://www.pubmedcentral.nih.gov/articlerender.fcgi?artid=3167817&tool=pmcentrez&rendertype=abstract

[19] Šmuc T, Ahn I-Y, Ulrich H. Nucleic acid aptamers as high affinity ligands in biotechnology and biosensorics. J Pharm Biomed Anal. 2013;81:210-7.

[20] Majumder P, Gomes KN, Ulrich H. Aptamers: from bench side research towards patented molecules with therapeutic applications. Expert Opin Ther Pat [Internet]. 2009 Nov 1;19(11):1603-13. Available from: https://doi.org/10.1517/13543770903313746

[21] Meek KN, Rangel AE, Heemstra JM. Enhancing aptamer function and stability via in vitro selection using modified nucleic acids. Methods. 2016 Aug;106:29-36.

[22] Kedzierski S, Khoshnejad M, Caltagirone GT. Synthetic antibodies: the emerging field of aptamers. Bioprocess J. 2012;11:46-9.

[23] Kaur H, Bruno JG, Kumar A, Sharma TK. Aptamers in the Therapeutics and Diagnostics Pipelines. Theranostics [Internet]. 2018 Jul 1;8(15):4016-32. Available from: https://pubmed.ncbi.nlm.nih.gov/30128033

[24] Ellington AD, Szostak JW. In vitro selection of RNA molecules that bind specific ligands. Nature. 1990;346(6287):818.

[25] Tuerk C, Gold L. Systematic evolution of ligands by exponential enrichment: RNA ligands to bacteriophage T4 DNA polymerase. Science. 1990;249(4968):505-10.

[26] Hofmann H-P, Limmer S, Hornung V, Sprinzl M. Ni2+-binding RNA motifs with an asymmetric purine-rich internal loop and a GA base pair. Rna. 1997;3(11):1289-300.

[27] Huizenga DE, Szostak JW. A DNA aptamer that binds adenosine and ATP. Biochemistry. 1995;34(2):656-65.

[28] Miyachi Y, Shimizu N, Ogino C, Fukuda H, Kondo A. Selection of a DNA aptamer that binds 8-OHdG using GMP-agarose. Bioorg Med Chem Lett. 2009;19(13):3619-22.

[29] Sett A, Borthakur BB, Sharma JD, Kataki AC, Bora U. DNA aptamer probes for detection of estrogen receptor α positive carcinomas. Transl Res. 2017;183:104-20.

[30] Sett A, Borthakur BB, Bora U. Selection of DNA aptamers for extra cellular domain of human epidermal growth factor receptor 2 to detect HER2 positive carcinomas. Clin Transl Oncol. 2017;19(8).

[31] Ahirwar R, Vellarikkal SK, Sett A, Sivasubbu S, Scaria V, Bora U, et al. Aptamer-Assisted Detection of the Altered Expression of Estrogen Receptor Alpha in Human Breast Cancer. PLoS One [Internet]. 2016;11(4):e0153001. Available from: http://journals.plos.org/plosone/article?id=10.1371/journal.pone.0153001

[32] Boese BJ, Breaker RR. In vitro selection and characterization of cellulose-binding DNA aptamers. Nucleic Acids Res. 2007;35(19):6378-88.

[33] Betat H, Vogel S, Struhalla M, Förster H-H, Famulok M, Welzel P, et al. Aptamers that recognize the lipid moiety of the antibiotic moenomycin A. Biol Chem. 2003;384(10-11):1497-500.

[34] Dwivedi HP, Smiley RD, Jaykus L-A. Selection and characterization of DNA aptamers with binding selectivity to

Campylobacter jejuni using whole-cell SELEX. Appl Microbiol Biotechnol. 2010;87(6):2323-34.

[35] Wang G, Liu J, Chen K, Xu Y, Liu B, Liao J, et al. Selection and characterization of DNA aptamer against glucagon receptor by cell-SELEX. Sci Rep. 2017;7(1):1-10.

[36] Pobanz K, Lupták A. Improving the odds: Influence of starting pools on in vitro selection outcomes. Methods. 2016;106:14-20.

[37] Stoltenburg R, Nikolaus N, Strehlitz B. Capture-SELEX: selection of DNA aptamers for aminoglycoside antibiotics. J Anal Methods Chem. 2012;2012.

[38] Paniel N, Istamboulié G, Triki A, Lozano C, Barthelmebs L, Noguer T. Selection of DNA aptamers against penicillin G using Capture-SELEX for the development of an impedimetric sensor. Talanta. 2017;162:232-40.

[39] Taylor AI, Houlihan G, Holliger P. Beyond DNA and RNA: The Expanding Toolbox of Synthetic Genetics. Cold Spring Harb Perspect Biol. 2019 Jun;11(6).

[40] Lee J, Schwieter KE, Watkins AM, Kim DS, Yu H, Schwarz KJ, et al. Expanding the limits of the second genetic code with ribozymes. Nat Commun. 2019 Nov;10(1):5097.

[41] Morihiro K, Kasahara Y, Obika S. Biological applications of xeno nucleic acids. Mol Biosyst. 2017 Jan;13(2):235-45.

[42] Rangel AE, Chen Z, Ayele TM, Heemstra JM. In vitro selection of an XNA aptamer capable of small-molecule recognition. Nucleic Acids Res. 2018;46(16).

[43] Vorobyeva MA, Davydova AS, Vorobjev PE, Venyaminova AG. Key Aspects of Nucleic Acid Library Design for in Vitro Selection. Int J Mol Sci [Internet]. 2018 Feb 5;19(2):470. Available from: https://pubmed.ncbi.nlm.nih.gov/29401748

[44] Jayasena SD. Aptamers: An emerging class of molecules that rival antibodies in diagnostics. Clin Chem. 1999;45(9):1628-50.

[45] Keefe AD, Pai S, Ellington A. Aptamers as therapeutics. Nat Rev Drug Discov [Internet]. 2010;9(7):537-50. Available from: http://dx.doi.org/10.1038/nrd3141

[46] Xiang D, Shigdar S, Qiao G, Wang T, Kouzani AZ, Zhou S-F, et al. Nucleic Acid Aptamer-Guided Cancer Therapeutics and Diagnostics: the Next Generation of Cancer Medicine. Theranostics [Internet]. 2015 Jan 1;5(1):23-42. Available from: http://www.ncbi.nlm.nih.gov/pmc/articles/PMC4265746/

[47] Cho EJ, Lee J-W, Ellington AD. Applications of aptamers as sensors. Annu Rev Anal Chem (Palo Alto Calif). 2009;2:241-64.

[48] Li S, Xu H, Ding H, Huang Y, Cao X, Yang G, et al. Identification of an aptamer targeting hnRNP A1 by tissue slide-based SELEX. 2009;(February):327-36.

[49] Autour A, Bouhedda F, Cubi R, Ryckelynck M. Optimization of fluorogenic RNA-based biosensors using droplet-based microfluidic ultrahigh-throughput screening. Methods. 2019;161:46-53.

[50] Barciszewski J, Medgaard M, Koch T, Kurreck J, Erdmann VA. Locked Nucleic Acid Aptamers. In: Nucleic Acid and Peptide Aptamers: Methods and Protocols [Internet]. 2009. p. 165-86. Available from: http://www.springerlink.com/index/10.1007/978-1-59745-557-2

[51] Veedu RN, Wengel J. Locked nucleic acids: promising nucleic acid analogs for therapeutic applications. Chem Biodivers. 2010;7(3):536-42.

[52] Darfeuille F, Hansen JB, Orum H, Di Primo C, Toulmé J-J. LNA/DNA chimeric oligomers mimic RNA aptamers targeted to the TAR RNA element of HIV-1. Nucleic Acids Res [Internet]. 2004 Jun 4;32(10):3101-7. Available from: https://www.ncbi.nlm.nih.gov/pubmed/15181175

[53] Langkjær N, Pasternak A, Wengel J. UNA (unlocked nucleic acid): a flexible RNA mimic that allows engineering of nucleic acid duplex stability. Bioorg Med Chem. 2009;17(15):5420-5.

[54] Wittung P, Nielsen PE, Buchardt O, Egholm M, Norde B. DNA-like double helix formed by peptide nucleic acid. Nature. 1994;368(6471):561-3.

[55] Floege J, Ostendorf T, Janssen U, Burg M, Radeke HH, Vargeese C, et al. Novel approach to specific growth factor inhibition in vivo: antagonism of platelet-derived growth factor in glomerulonephritis by aptamers. Am J Pathol. 1999;154(1):169-79.

[56] Santosh B, Yadava PK. Nucleic Acid Aptamers: Research Tools in Disease Diagnostics and Therapeutics. Biomed Res Int [Internet]. 2014;2014:1-13. Available from: http://www.pubmedcentral.nih.gov/articlerender.fcgi?artid=4090538&tool=pmcentrez&rendertype=abstract

[57] Ruckman J, Green LS, Beeson J, Waugh S, Gillette WL, Henninger DD, et al. 2′-Fluoropyrimidine RNA-based aptamers to the 165-amino acid form of vascular endothelial growth factor (VEGF165) inhibition of receptor binding and VEGF-induced vascular permeability through interactions requiring the exon 7-encoded domain. J Biol Chem. 1998;273(32):20556-67.

[58] Lee J-H, Canny MD, De Erkenez A, Krilleke D, Ng Y-S, Shima DT, et al. A therapeutic aptamer inhibits angiogenesis by specifically targeting the heparin binding domain of VEGF165. Proc Natl Acad Sci. 2005;102(52):18902-7.

[59] Lipi F, Chen S, Chakravarthy M, Rakesh S, Veedu RN. In vitro evolution of chemically-modified nucleic acid aptamers: Pros and cons, and comprehensive selection strategies. RNA Biol [Internet]. 2016 Dec 1;13(12):1232-45. Available from: https://doi.org/10.1080/15476286.2016.1236173

[60] Kimoto M, Matsunaga K, Hirao I. Evolving Aptamers with Unnatural Base Pairs. Curr Protoc Chem Biol. 2017;9(4):315-39.

[61] Ng EWM, Shima DT, Calias P, Cunningham ET, Guyer DR, Adamis AP. Pegaptanib, a targeted anti-VEGF aptamer for ocular vascular disease. Nat Rev Drug Discov. 2006;5(2):123-32.

[62] Sampson T. Aptamers and SELEX: The technology. World Pat Inf. 2003;25(2):123-9.

[63] Shamah SM, Healy JM, Cload ST. Complex target SELEX. Acc Chem Res. 2008;41(1):130-8.

[64] Lao Y-H, Phua KKL, Leong KW. Aptamer nanomedicine for cancer therapeutics: barriers and potential for translation. ACS Nano. 2015;9(3):2235-54.

[65] Carvalho J, Paiva A, Campello MPC, Paulo A, Mergny J-L, Salgado GF, et al. Aptamer-based targeted Delivery of a G-quadruplex Ligand in Cervical Cancer Cells. Sci Rep. 2019;9(1):1-12.

[66] Rosenberg JE, Bambury RM, Van Allen EM, Drabkin HA, Lara PN, Harzstark AL, et al. A phase II trial of AS1411 (a novel nucleolin-targeted DNA aptamer) in metastatic renal

cell carcinoma. Invest New Drugs. 2014;32(1):178-87.

[67] Hoellenriegel J, Zboralski D, Maasch C, Rosin NY, Wierda WG, Keating MJ, et al. The Spiegelmer NOX-A12, a novel CXCL12 inhibitor, interferes with chronic lymphocytic leukemia cell motility and causes chemosensitization. Blood. 2014;123(7):1032-9.

[68] Kruschinski MGSC-CMJTDZZR. Anti-CXCL12/SDF-1 Spiegelmer® Nox-A12 alone and in combination with bendamustine and rituximab in patients with relapsed chronic lymphocytic leukemia (CLL): results from a phase IIa study [Abstract 1635]. 55th American Society of Hematology Annual Meeting and Exhibition. 2013.

[69] Pestourie C, Tavitian B, Duconge F. Aptamers against extracellular targets for in vivo applications. Biochimie. 2005;87(9-10):921-30.

[70] Zhou J, Rossi JJ. Cell-specific aptamer-mediated targeted drug delivery. Oligonucleotides. 2011;21(1):1-10.

[71] Li N, Nguyen HH, Byrom M, Ellington AD. Inhibition of cell proliferation by an anti-EGFR aptamer. PLoS One. 2011;6(6):e20299.

[72] Hicke BJ, Stephens AW. Escort aptamers: a delivery service for diagnosis and therapy. J Clin Invest. 2000;106(8):923-8.

[73] Gijs M, Aerts A, Impens N, Baatout S, Luxen A. Aptamers as radiopharmaceuticals for nuclear imaging and therapy. Nucl Med Biol. 2016;43(4):253-71.

[74] Inkster JAH, Adam MJ, Storr T, Ruth TJ. Labeling of an antisense oligonucleotide with [18F] FPy5yne. Nucleosides, Nucleotides and Nucleic Acids. 2009;28(11-12):1131-43.

[75] Mercier F, Paris J, Kaisin G, Thonon D, Flagothier J, Teller N, et al. General method for labeling siRNA by click chemistry with fluorine-18 for the purpose of PET imaging. Bioconjug Chem. 2011;22(1):108-14.

[76] Lange CW, VanBrocklin HF, Taylor SE. Photoconjugation of 3-azido-5-nitrobenzyl-[18F] fluoride to an oligonucleotide aptamer. J Label Compd Radiopharm. 2002;45(3):257-68.

[77] Bandekar A, Zhu C, Jindal R, Bruchertseifer F, Morgenstern A, Sofou S. Anti–prostate-specific membrane antigen liposomes loaded with 225Ac for potential targeted antivascular α-particle therapy of cancer. J Nucl Med. 2014;55(1):107-14.

[78] Charlton J, Sennello J, Smith D. In vivo imaging of inflammation using an aptamer inhibitor of human neutrophil elastase. Chem Biol. 1997;4(11):809-16.

[79] Hicke BJ, Marion C, Chang Y-F, Gould T, Lynott CK, Parma D, et al. Tenascin-C aptamers are generated using tumor cells and purified protein. J Biol Chem. 2001;276(52):48644-54.

[80] Hicke BJ, Stephens AW, Gould T, Chang Y-F, Lynott CK, Heil J, et al. Tumor targeting by an aptamer. J Nucl Med. 2006;47(4):668-78.

[81] Ouellet J. RNA Fluorescence with Light-Up Aptamers. Front Chem [Internet]. 2016;4(June):1-12.

[82] Bouhedda F, Autour A, Ryckelynck M. Light-up RNA aptamers and their cognate fluorogens: from their development to their applications. Int J Mol Sci. 2018;19(1):44.

[83] Sett A, Zara L, Dausse E, Toulme J-J. Engineering light-up aptamers for the detection of RNA hairpins through kissing interaction. Anal Chem. 2020 Jun 4;0(ja).

[84] Durand G, Lisi S, Ravelet C, Dausse E, Peyrin E, Toulmé JJ. Riboswitches based on kissing complexes for the detection of small ligands. Angew Chemie - Int Ed. 2014;53(27):6942-5.

[85] Germer K, Leonard M, Zhang X. RNA aptamers and their therapeutic and diagnostic applications. Vol. 4, International Journal of Biochemistry and Molecular Biology. 2013. p. 27-40.

[86] Tan W, Wang H, Chen Y, Zhang X, Zhu H, Yang C, et al. Molecular aptamers for drug delivery. Trends Biotechnol. 2011;29(12):634-40.

Chapter 4

Extracellular Vesicles: "Stealth Transport Aircrafts" for Drugs

Chunying Liu, Xuejing Lin and Changqing Su

Abstract

Extracellular vesicles (EVs) can deliver many types of drugs with their natural source material transport properties, inherent long-term blood circulation capabilities and excellent biocompatibility, and have great potential in the field of drug carrier. Modification of the content and surface of EVs according to the purpose of treatment has become a research focus to improve the drug load and the targeting of EVs. EVs can maximize the stability of the drugs, prevent immune clearance and achieve accurate delivery. Therefore, EVs can be described as "stealth transport aircrafts" for drugs. This chapter will respectively introduce the application of natural EVs as cell substitutes in cell therapy and engineered EVs as carriers of nucleic acids, proteins, small molecule drugs and therapeutic viral particles in disease treatment. It will also explain the drug loading and modification strategies of EVs, the source and characteristics of EVs. In addition, the commercialization progress of EVs drugs will be mentioned here, and the problems in their applications will be discussed in conjunction with the application of EVs in the treatment of COVID-19.

Keywords: extracellular vesicles, exosomes, drug carrier, drug loading, targeting modification

1. Introduction

Extracellular vesicles (EVs) are a collective term for tiny vesicles with a phospholipid bilayer structure that are actively secreted by cells. Almost all known cell types can be secreted. The two main categories of EVs are exosomes and microvesicles (**Table 1**). Exosomes (30-150 nm in diameter) are intraluminal vesicles, formed by the invagination of the multivesicular endosome membrane, and are released into the extracellular space after the multivesicular endosomes fuse with the cell membrane [1]. Microvesicles (50–1,000 nm in diameter) are a group of highly heterogeneous EVs characterized in that their origin and secretion are budding through the plasma membrane [1]. Considering the complexity of identifying its biogenesis, the size of the vesicle is the most widely used parameter for classifying EV types,

Vesicle	Size (nm)	Density (g/mL)	Origin	Markers
Exosomes	30-150	1.13-1.18	Endosomes	Tetraspanins, Alix, TSG101
Microvesicles	50-1000	1.16-1.19	Plasma membrane	Intergrins, Selectins, CD40

Table 1.
The main characteristics of EVs [1, 2].

and on this basis they are described as small EVs or medium and large EVs. In this article, unless otherwise specified, the term "EVs" generally refers to small EVs.

In recent years, people's understanding of the biogenesis, composition, function and mechanism of EVs has continued to deepen [3–5]. Their application in clinical treatment has also attracted more and more attention. One of the most useful properties of EVs is their ability to cross barriers, such as the plasma membrane and blood/brain barrier. This makes them very suitable for delivering therapeutic molecules. With their natural source material transport properties, inherent long-term blood circulation capabilities and excellent biocompatibility, EVs can deliver a variety of chemical drugs, proteins, nucleic acids, gene drugs and other drugs. They have great potential in the field of drug carriers. CD47 is the ligand for signal regulatory protein alpha (SIRPα), and CD47-SIRPα binding initiates the 'don't eat me' signal that inhibits phagocytosis. Therefore, CD47 on EVs prevents them from being engulfed by immune cells [6]. EVs are more efficient than their synthetic analog liposomes. The application of EVs as drug delivery carriers is like putting a "stealth coat" on the drug molecules, which can maximize the stability of the drugs, reduce the immune system's clearance of them, and make "precise delivery" possible. Therefore, EVs can be described as "stealth transport aircrafts" for drugs. EVs therapy has shown great application prospects from oncology to regenerative medicine.

2. Therapeutic application of natural EVs as cell substitutes

A number of studies have shown that EVs derived from mesenchymal stem cells (MSCs) can be used for stem cell replacement therapy [7–21]. In most cases, it is not clear which component of the unmodified EVs exerts curative effects. The researchers' operations are only the separation and purification of EVs produced by therapeutic cells. The curative effects are based on the biological functions of the donor cells, such as the regulation of the immune environment, the repair of damaged cells and the promotion of angiogenesis.

At present, the most extensive research is the attempt to use stem cell-derived EVs for disease treatment. The main application ranges are to repair and regenerate tissues and organs. Such researches involve central nervous system diseases [7, 8], cardiovascular diseases [9–12] and other organ damage repair and regeneration [13–21].

2.1 EVs derived from stem cells and the treatment of central nervous system diseases

In the treatment of central nervous system disease, there is a blood-brain barrier, which often results in that drugs can not reach the diseased site and work well. Stem cells have been gradually used in the treatment of central nervous system diseases in recent years. A large number of research results have been obtained [22, 23]. However, there are still potential risks faced by direct stem cell transplantation, such as tumorigenicity, infection, transplant failure, graft versus host disease, hemorrhagic cystitis, and long-term complications [24].

The application of stem cell EVs avoids a variety of potential risks of direct stem cell transplantation. EVs have low immunogenicity and are easy to preserve and transport, showing unique advantages as a "cell-free stem cell therapy technology". Spinal cord injury (SCI) is one of the deadliest diseases. The complex inhibitory microenvironment needs to be fully mitigated. EVs derived from MSCs have the function of microenvironmental regulation. Studies have established innovative implantation strategies using human MSC-derived EVs immobilized in peptide-modified adhesive hydrogels (Exo-pGel) [7]. Exo-pGel plays an important role in nerve recovery and urinary tissue protection by effectively reducing inflammation and oxidation [7]. In addition, small extracellular vesicles derived from embryonic stem cells (ESC-sEVs) can significantly reduce the time-related aging of hippocampal neural stem cells (H-NSCs) through intravenous injection into vascular dementia (VD) rats. ESC-sEVs can restore the damaged proliferation and neuronal differentiation ability, and reverse cognitive impairment. The application of ESC-sEVs may be a new cell-free treatment tool for VD and other diseases related to aging [8].

2.2 EVs derived from stem cells and the treatment of cardiovascular diseases

Stem cells can be induced to differentiate into cardiomyocytes. Early studies believed that the transplanted stem cells can differentiate into heart cells and necrotic cells in the body to repair damaged myocardium and maintain heart function [25]. At present, a large number of preclinical studies have found that EVs derived from transplanted stem cells also have the function of myocardial repair [26, 27]. EVs mainly promote myocardial regeneration by activating cardiac precursor cells, promoting the survival and proliferation of cardiomyocytes, inhibiting their apoptosis, promoting cardiac angiogenesis, reducing infarct size and tissue fibrosis, and regulating inflammation. Extracellular vesicles secreted by cardiovascular precursor cells (hCVPC-EVs) derived from human pluripotent stem cells (hPSCs) play a role in protecting the heart in myocardial infarction by improving cardiomyocyte survival and angiogenesis [9]. Mouse ESC-derived EVs promote angiogenesis, cardiomyocyte survival and proliferation, reduce cardiac fibrosis, and improve cardiac function by carrying miR-294-3p [10]. IPSC-derived EVs inhibit cardiomyocyte apoptosis through miR-21 and miR-210 loaded, and also have a cardioprotective effect [11]. Exosomes produced by immature bone marrow-derived macrophages (BMDM-exo) contain anti-inflammatory microRNA-99a/146b/378a. They can reduce the necrotic lesions of atherosclerosis [12].

2.3 EVs derived from stem cells and the damage repair and regeneration of other organs

With the continuous discovery of the repair and regeneration effects of stem cell EVs in brain tissue and cardiovascular tissues and organs, the application of stem cell EVs in the repair and regeneration of other tissues has also made a lot of progresses.

MSC-derived EVs reduce radiation-induced lung injury through miRNA-214-3p [13]. Replacing autologous cells with EVs derived from hair follicle papillary cell spheres can promote hair growth [14]. Human umbilical cord mesenchymal stem cell-derived exosomes (UMSC-Exo) can inhibit pyrolysis and repair muscle ischemic injury by releasing circular RNA circHIPK3 [15]. Hertwig's EVs derived from epithelial root sheath cells promote the regeneration of dentin plasma tissue [16]. Exosomes from neural progenitor cells retain photoreceptor cells during retinal degeneration (RD) by inactivating microglia. This suggests that NPC-exos and its contents may be the mechanism of stem cell therapy to treat RD [17].

Aging is the process of cell and tissue dysfunction. Small extracellular vesicles (sEVs) isolated from primary fibroblasts from young human donors can improve certain biomarkers of cellular senescence from elderly and Hutchinson-Gilford progeria donors. Studies have shown that sEVs have GST activity to improve aging-related tissue damage [18]. In obesity diseases, EVs derived from adipocytes, as new adipokines, are related to the body's metabolic homeostasis. EVs released from brown adipose tissue or adipose stem cells can help control the remodeling of white adipose tissue, making it brown and maintaining metabolic homeostasis. EVs have been considered as new regulators of diseases such as insulin resistance, diabetes and non-alcoholic fatty liver. The results provide new treatment strategies for obesity and metabolic diseases [19].

In addition, some reports suggest that some EVs derived from mesenchymal stem cells contain some tumor suppressor molecules. For example, it has been reported that miR-206 in exosomes derived from bone marrow mesenchymal stem cells could inhibit the progression of osteosarcoma by targeting TRA2B [20]. The exosomes derived from human umbilical cord mesenchymal stem cells deliver miRNA-375 to delay the progression of esophageal squamous cell carcinoma [21]. However, although EVs contain these small RNAs that have been reported to exert anti-cancer effects, they also contain a large number of growth factors and pro-angiogenesis factors. When these substances are transported to tumor cells by EVs, can EVs derived from MSCs still exert a tumor suppressor effect? This needs more research to prove.

At present, cell replacement therapy based on the characteristics of donor cells has been studied earlier and more frequently in the field of EVs. There is also a clearer understanding of the components that play a major role. With the continuous increase of clinical needs, people began to try to modify the surfaces and contents of EVs to adapt to more disease treatments.

3. Application of engineered EVs as carriers of nucleic acid drugs in disease treatment

Although natural EVs have been used for cell replacement therapy based on their source and achieved good results, their therapeutic range is far from meeting the current treatment needs. One of the most important therapeutic areas is the treatment of malignant tumors. The secretion ability of EVs in malignant tumor itself is enhanced and contributes to tumor progression. Considering that MSC-derived EVs generally contain high levels of growth factors and pro-angiogenic factors, most natural EVs are not suitable for tumor therapy, except that EVs derived from antigen-presenting cells can be used as tumor vaccines to activate anti-tumor immune responses [28]. Based on the biological characteristics of EVs, it has become the focus of researchers and biopharmaceutical companies to transform EVs as carriers of multiple drugs.

Most diseases have characteristic down-regulation of small RNA expression. Small RNA is the main content of extracellular vesicles, the most abundant and the most easily carried component. Therefore, EVs can be used to carry and deliver small RNA and other gene therapy systems. This section will discuss the progress of engineered EVs to deliver nucleic acid drugs and the strategies of drug loading and targeting.

3.1 Research progress of engineered EVs to deliver nucleic acid drugs

There are three main problems in the development of nucleic acid drugs: the instability of nucleic acid molecules in the body, potential side effects and difficulties in drug delivery systems. The most important one is the development of delivery systems. Because a good drug delivery system can improve drug stability and target cell absorption efficiency, and can reduce its side effects. At present, the commonly used delivery vehicles in the field of nucleic acid drugs are mainly adeno-associated virus (AAV) and liposomal nanoparticles (LNPs). A small number of companies also use lentivirus (LV) and exosomes as delivery vehicles.

The packaging capacity of AAV is small (≤5kb). AAV will be used more than once in patients for therapeutic purposes and the second use will cause the body to produce a strong immune response. The safety of LNPs is relatively high, and the carrier capacity and delivery efficiency can meet the current demand for drug carriers. However, the organ selectivity of LNPs is still relatively limited. The main delivery area is concentrated in the liver, and the delivery efficiency to other tissues and organs is relatively low.

EVs are now candidate carriers for nucleic acid drugs by virtue of their advantages. The red blood cell extracellular vesicles (RBCEVs) have a large loading capacity (≤11kb), can be loaded with many types (including DNA, mRNA, antisense oligonucleotides, siRNA and other nucleic acid types), and contain very little nucleic acid. The advantages make them high-quality natural blank nucleic acid carriers. RBCEVs can be delivered to many different organs and tissues. In mouse experiments, the delivery effects of lung, liver, kidney, bone tissue, immune cells, etc. are all obvious [29]. Moreover, the raw materials used to produce RBCEVs are mainly blood from type O blood donors. This means large quantities of raw materials are readily available, and costs are controllable. Carmine Therapeutics focuses on the research and development of nucleic acid delivery technology using RBCEVs as carriers.

In addition, researchers are also committed to modifying the surfaces of EVs to improve their targeting. Many results show that this strategy can indeed improve the therapeutic effect of engineered EVs [30–33].

The researchers combined ligand-coupled superparamagnetic nanoparticles with specific membrane proteins of blood exosomes to achieve the separation, purification and tumor targeting of exosomes [30]. The chemotherapy drug doxorubicin (Dox) and the cholesterol-modified single-stranded miRNA-21 inhibitor (chol-miR21i) were co-loaded onto the exosomes. Then the cationic endolysin peptide was absorbed on the negatively charged membrane surface of exosomes to promote the cytoplasmic release of the packaged cargo (**Figure 1**). The research results showed that these effectively released drugs and RNA simultaneously interfered with nuclear DNA activity and down-regulated the expression of oncogenes, thereby significantly inhibiting tumor growth and reducing side effects [30].

Chimeric antigen receptors (CAR) are cell surface receptors that recognize specific proteins (antigens). Tumor cells express their specific antigens. Modification of EVs surfaces with CAR targeting tumor antigens enables EVs to target tumors for

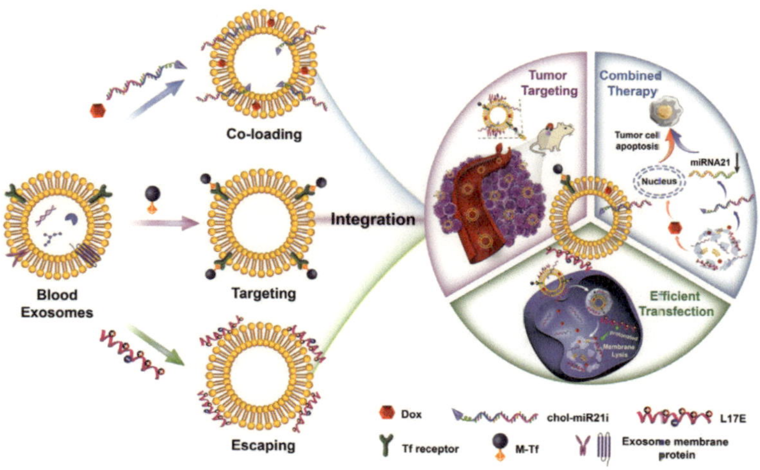

Figure 1.
Schematic representation of engineered blood exosomes for effective gene/chemo combined antitumor therapy [30].

drug delivery. Modified EVs with CAR can serve as a biosafety delivery platform for the CRISPR/Cas9 system to improve their tumor selectivity. Compared with unmodified EVs, CAR-EVs accumulate rapidly in tumors and effectively release the CRISPR/Cas9 system targeting MYC oncogenes in vitro and in vivo [31].

Rabies virus glycoprotein (RVG) is neurogenic. At present, it has become the most active guide molecule for brain targeted drugs. Lysosomal-associated membrane glycoprotein 2b (Lamp2b) is the membrane surface protein of EVs. RVG fused with Lamp2b is located on the surface of the EV to achieve brain targeting. Engineered Lamp2b-RVG-circSCMH1-extracellular vesicles (Lamp2b-RVG-circSCMH1-EVs) can selectively deliver circSCMH1 to the brain. The treatment can improve the functional recovery of mice and monkeys after stroke [32].

In addition, EVs without modification for targeting have also shown certain curative effects. The miR-214 inhibitor was transfected into HEK293T cells. Their exosomes Exo-anti-214 can reverse the resistance of gastric cancer to DDP [33]. HEK293T cells were transfected with HGF siRNA and their exosomes were harvested. In vivo and in vitro experiments have shown that exosomes loaded with HGF siRNA can inhibit the proliferation and migration of cancer cells and vascular cells [33].

3.2 Methods of loading nucleic acid drugs into engineered EVs

Methods of loading nucleic acids into EVs include: chemical reagent transfection, electroporation transfection, transfection of donor cells, protein and characteristic sequence targeting methods. The application scope and advantages and disadvantages of different methods are shown in **Table 2**.

The use of proteins that can bind to specific RNA sequences (**Figure 2**) or the conservative sequences of Exosome-enriched RNAs (eRNAs) to achieve active packaging is a promising direction. The researchers used the specificity of protein binding to the RNA sequence to develop EXOtic devices for mRNA delivery [38]. Archaeal ribosomal protein L7Ae specifically binds to the C/Dbox RNA structure [40–42]. Based on this, L7Ae was conjugated to the C-terminus of CD63. C/D box

Methods	Application scope	Merit and demerit	References
Chemical reagent transfection	Broad-spectrum.	Easy to operate, but EVs should be purified before and after transfection.	[34]
Electroporation transfection	The most commonly used method, but not for miRNA, shRNA, mRNA containing chemical modification.	Easy to operate, but EVs should be purified before and after transfection.	[35]
Transfection of donor cells	Broad spectrum, but not for biotoxic molecules.	Purify EVs after transfection, but the effect of the transfected molecule on the donor cell should be taken into account (e.g. biotoxicity).	[33, 36, 37]
Protein and characteristic sequence targeting	mRNA and miRNA.	High specificity of loading, but the therapeutic molecules will be modified. Whether this will affect the efficacy remains to be determined.	[38, 39]

Table 2.
Methods of loading nucleic acid drugs into engineered EVs.

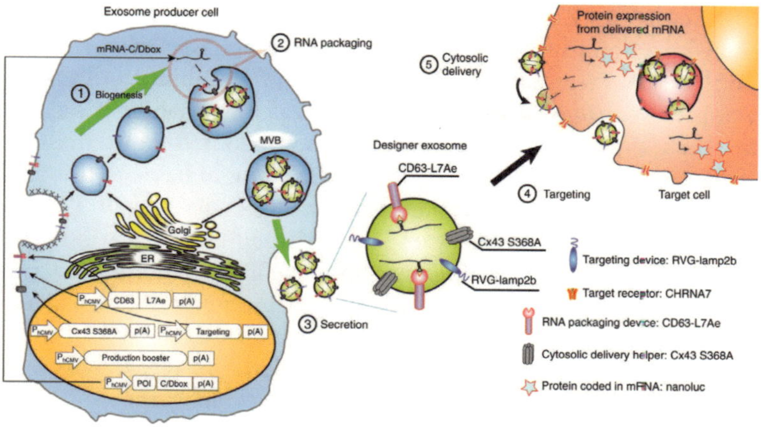

Figure 2.
EXOtic devices for mRNA delivery. A schematic illustration of the EXOtic devices [38].

was inserted into the 3′-untranslated region (3′-UTR) of the reporter gene. Therefore, the mRNA encoding the reporter protein could be well incorporated into exosomes via the interaction between L7Ae and the C/D box in the 3′-UTR. Exosomes containing the RNA packaging device (CD63-L7Ae), targeting module (RVG-Lamp2b to target CHRNA7), cytosolic delivery helper (Cx43 S368A) and mRNA (nluc-C/Dbox) were efficiently produced from exosome producer cells by the exosome production booster. The engineered exosomes were delivered to target cells and the mRNA was delivered into the target cell cytosol with the help of the cytosolic delivery helper. Finally, protein encoded in the mRNA was expressed in the target cells [38] (**Figure 2**). In the future, researchers need to obtain more specific RNA sequence binding proteins and conserved sequences of eRNAs through bioinformatics analysis.

4. Application of engineered EVs as protein transporters in disease treatment

The lack of protein and malfunction are important causes of many diseases. For example, the occurrence of malignant tumors is related to the lack of certain tumor suppressor factors and malfunctions. Therefore, increasing the corresponding protein level is one of the ways to treat diseases. Considering the risk of genome changes, researchers aim to deliver therapeutic protein molecules to the lesion through effective drug delivery vehicles. This section will introduce the use of EVs to transport protein molecules for the prevention and treatment of tumors, immune diseases, cardiovascular diseases, atherosclerosis, myocardial infarction and other diseases.

4.1 Research progress of engineered EVs as protein transporters for disease treatment

Compared with the previous small molecule compound drugs, protein drugs have the characteristics of high activity, strong specificity, low toxicity, clear biological functions, and are beneficial to clinical application. However, protein drugs are unstable in the internal and external environments, and may undergo a variety of complex chemical degradation and physical changes, such as aggregation, precipitation, racemization, hydrolysis, and deamidation. Protein drugs have short half-life, high clearance rate, large molecular weight, poor permeability, susceptibility to the destruction of enzymes, bacteria and body fluids in the receptor, and low bioavailability of non-injection administration. These problems greatly limit the use of protein drugs. Although researchers have improved the stability and absorption efficiency of protein drugs through methods such as PEG modification, microsphere sustained release, and liposome embedding, they still look forward to the emergence of better drug carriers. The application of EVs has brought dawn to this field.

Tumor necrosis factor (TNF)-related apoptosis-inducing ligand (TRAIL) is a promising anticancer agent. Delivery of TRAIL through EVs can efficiently induce cancer cell apoptosis. When combined with dinaciclib, they inhibit the growth of drug-resistant tumors [43]. Immunosuppressive drugs must be taken after organ transplantation, but long-term use of these drugs increases the risk of infection and other serious diseases. Using bioengineering methods, researchers prepared exosome-like nanovesicles (NV) displaying the dual target cargo of PD-L1/CTLA-4. These NVs enhanced the PD-L1/PD-1 and CTLA-4/CD80 immunosuppressive pathways and could be used as prospective immunosuppressive agents in organ transplantation [44]. Using extracellular nanovesicles to package CRISPR-Cas9 protein and sgRNA to induce therapeutic exon skipping can avoid off-target mutagenesis and immunogenicity. And this method can achieve effective genome editing in a variety of cell types that are difficult to transfect, including human induced pluripotent stem cells (iPS), neurons and myoblasts [45]. Catalase could be loaded into exosomes by incubating at room temperature, saponins penetrating the membrane, repeated freezing and thawing and mechanical extrusion for the treatment of Parkinson's disease (PD) [46].

Surface modification of EVs carrying protein drugs can greatly improve their targeting. In the study of stroke, nerve growth factor (NGF) exerts various neuroprotective functions after ischemia. NGF was loaded into EVs with RVG peptide modification on the surface. Through systemic administration, NGF was effectively delivered to the ischemic cortex. The delivered NGF reduced inflammation by remodeling microglia polarization, promoted cell survival, and increased the number of neuroblast marker doublecortin-positive cells. The results of the study indicated the potential therapeutic effect of NGF@Exo (RVG) on stroke [47]. In addition, integrin $\alpha V\beta 5$ exhibits tropism for the liver while integrin $\alpha 6V\beta 4$ and integrin $\alpha 6\beta 1$ target lung [48, 49]. The iRGD specifically recognizes αV integrins on the surface of tumor cells [50]. RVG and c(RGDyK) peptides target brain tissue [51]. Klotho protein has the property of binding to circulating endothelial progenitor cells (EPCs) [52]. And chimeric antigen receptor (CAR) targeting specific tumor antigens and so on. These guiding molecules are utilized either by fusion with EVs membrane surface proteins (such as Lamp2b, VSVG, CD63, and other transmembrane proteins, etc.), or by chemical cross-linking on the surface of EVs to achieve the EVs targeting modification. Liu et al. summarized the surface modification strategies to improve the targeting of EVs (**Figure 3**) [53]. In addition, EVs derived from antigen-presenting cells with tumor antigens can be used as tumor vaccines to activate anti-tumor immune responses.

4.2 Methods of loading protein drugs into EVs

How to load protein drugs into EVs? There are currently the following strategies:

4.2.1 Expression of therapeutic protein in donor cells

Transfect donor cells with plasmids carrying the gene of interest. The cell will synthesize the target protein. These proteins are then secreted into EVs through a

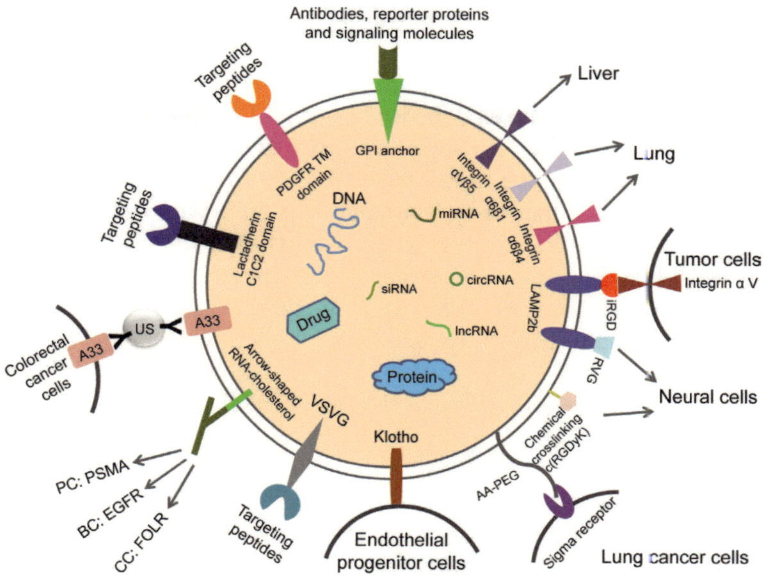

Figure 3.
Design strategies for therapeutic exosome targeting [53].

natural packaging process. Subsequent separation and purification of EVs in the cell culture supernatant is sufficient [54]. Although this method seems simple and easy to implement, cytotoxicity, mixed interactions and impaired biological responses will provide great obstacles to the production of EVs. And the loading efficiency of the target protein is relatively low. Therefore, researchers have carried out various attempts to specifically load target proteins into EVs. For example, the fusion of therapeutic proteins with the constituent proteins of EVs and the specific modification of therapeutic proteins.

4.2.2 Fusion of therapeutic protein with the constituent proteins of EVs

The therapeutic proteins are fused with the constituent proteins of EVs. Then they will be distributed into EVs mediated by the constituent proteins. This method can improve the specificity of protein loading into EVs. The fused constituent proteins of EVs that have been tried include: CD63, Nef [55], vesicular stomatitis virus glycoprotein (VSVG) [56], apolipoprotein E (ApoE) [57], lysosome-associated membrane glycoprotein 2 (LAMP2B) [58], etc.

In addition, based on the idea of fusion proteins, researchers have developed a conditional loading method called "exosomes for protein loading via optically reversible protein-protein interaction (EXPLORs)" [59]. The principle is to couple the exosomal membrane protein CD9 with CIBN, and CRY 2 with the therapeutic protein. After light excitation, CIBN and CRY2 interact, and the therapeutic protein can be loaded into EVs through "photoreversible protein-protein interaction" [59].

All in all, the fusion expression of therapeutic proteins with the constituent proteins of EVs can indeed increase the enrichment level of therapeutic proteins in EVs. However, whether the fusion protein affects the uptake and function of the therapeutic protein by the recipient cells needs to be verified. Therefore, exploring the fusion of peptides that can play a sorting role with therapeutic proteins and minimize the impact on protein functions will become one of the research hotspots in the field of engineered EVs.

4.2.3 Specific modification of therapeutic protein

Currently, known protein modifications that can target therapeutic proteins into EVs mainly include two types. One is ubiquitination modification. The fusion of ubiquitin to the C-terminus of therapeutic protein can make the concentration of the fused therapeutic protein in EVs increased by nearly 10 times [60]. The other is to fuse the N-terminus of the therapeutic protein with a palmitoylated or myristoylated peptide, which can further increase the therapeutic protein in EVs [61]. However, it is still unknown whether the modification of proteins, especially ubiquitination, will cause the degradation of the therapeutic protein by the proteasome and affect its function in the recipient cell.

4.2.4 Combined with mechanical methods to produce small vesicles containing therapeutic proteins

Expression of therapeutic protein in donor cells, combined with mechanical methods that pass through different pores, can produce small vesicles containing the therapeutic proteins [46, 62]. In addition, there are methods such as incubation at room temperature, permeabilization with saponin, freeze-thaw cycles and sonication, [46]. There are two main problems with engineered EVs obtained by mechanical methods. One is that the technical requirements for the separation and purification of EVs are relatively high. The second is the maintenance of the integrity and biological activity of EVs. The composition of EVs actively produced by cells is different from the composition of mechanically produced EVs. The difference may affect the efficacy of engineered EVs. In the future application research of EVs, these two problems need to be solved and proved urgently.

So, what are the possible development directions for the existing cytotoxicity and the interaction of biological functions? The expression of tumor suppressor protein molecules may cause cytotoxicity to donor cells, which is not conducive to the production of EVs. If an inducible expression system is established, the coding DNA containing the inducible promoter is introduced into the donor cell to make the donor cell produce EVs containing the coding DNA, which will avoid cytotoxicity to the donor cell. Then prepare EVs containing small molecules that induce DNA expression. The two types of EVs can be used in combination to express tumor suppressor molecules in target cells. It can play a therapeutic role without affecting the production efficiency of EVs. The dual targeting of the two EVs will greatly reduce the impact of engineered EVs on non-targeted tissues. Because single-component EVs are randomly engulfed by cells and will not affect the cells. This may become one of the follow-up development directions in this field.

5. Application of engineered EVs as carriers of small compounds in disease treatment

Chemotherapeutics and traditional Chinese medicine ingredients with anticancer effects are often used in the clinical treatment of a variety of malignant tumors. However, their toxic, side effects and short half-life limit their efficacy. The packaging and transportation with EVs will improve the targeting of chemotherapeutic drugs, increase the uptake efficiency of tumor cells, promote drug stability, reduce the use concentration, and reduce toxic side effects on other organs and normal tissues [63].

The hydrophobic drug curcumin could be packaged into exosomes by direct mixing for tumor treatment [64]. Paclitaxel (PTX) was loaded into EVs secreted by macrophages by different methods such as room temperature incubation, electroporation and sonication. Studies have found that ultrasound treatment increases the load of EVs on drug molecules and the sustained release [65]. Small compounds can also be naturally secreted into EVs by incubating with donor cells. Incubation with paclitaxel make mesenchymal stromal cells produce microvesicles containing paclitaxel [66]. Injecting methotrexate-containing plasma membrane microvesicles (MTX-TMP) from apoptotic human tumor cells into the bile duct lumen of extrahepatic CCA patients could mobilize and activate neutrophils, and relieve the bile duct obstruction in 25% of patients, almost no adverse reactions [67].

At present, small molecule drugs are often loaded into EVs by passive loading methods, such as direct mixing, incubation, ultrasonic treatment, vortexing, saponin permeation, repeated freezing and thawing, and mechanical extrusion. The disadvantages of these methods have always existed, that is, the loss and quality reduction of EVs caused by multiple purifications. In addition, long-term in vitro processing and the physical and chemical properties of drug molecules will also affect the biological activity and stability of EVs. Therefore, before EVs can be widely used in treatment, the storage methods and stability factors of EVs are also worthy of research.

6. Application of engineered EVs as virus carriers in gene therapy

Why are EVs a "stealth cap" for drugs? Because we know viruses to use them exactly like this. In nature, viruses "hijack" EVs to secrete and infect other cells. This method helps to provide a "cover" for the virus to prevent the virus from being cleared by the immune system or neutralized by antibodies, such as the infection process of HAV, HBV and HCV.

In gene therapy, currently widely used adeno-associated virus (AAV), oncolytic adenovirus (OAV) and lentivirus (LV) mediated gene therapy can cause the body's immune response. After the same kind of AAV is used once, the body will produce a strong immune response, making the second injection ineffective. If EVs encapsulate viral particles to mediate their delivery, perhaps the therapeutic effect will be better.

Studies have shown that AAV isolated from conditioned media could bind to exosomes (exo-AAV) [68]. Compared with conventional AAV, exo-AAV was more resistant to neutralizing antibodies. After systemic injection in mice, compared with conventional AAV, exo-AAV delivered genes to the brain more efficiently at low vector doses. Importantly, no cytotoxicity was found in exo-AAV transduced cells. This may make exo-AAV widely used as a neuroscience research tool [68]. Compared with non-targeted modified EV-AAV, the expression of brain-targeting peptides on the surfaces of EVs can significantly enhance transduction [69].

In gene therapy of ophthalmic diseases, transferring genes to the retina is challenging. Because it requires a carrier system to overcome physical and biochemical barriers to enter and spread throughout the retinal tissue. After the exo-AAV was injected into the vitreous cavity (IVT), it was found that the expression of exo-AAV was better than the traditional AAV. Exo-AAV exhibited a deeper penetration in the retina, effectively reaching the inner core and outer plexus, and to a lesser extent the outer nuclear layer. Exo-AAV is a reliable mouse retina gene delivery tool. Its simplicity of production and isolation makes it widely used in basic eye research [70].

Due to the low efficiency of gene delivery to the inner ear sensory hair cells. AAV is not so advanced in the field of gene therapy for hearing impairment. Studies have shown that Exo-AAV1-GFP is more effective than traditional AAV1-GFP, whether injected in mouse cochlear explants in vitro or directly injected into the cochlea in vivo. Exo-AAV was not toxic in the body. Exo-AAV1 gene therapy partially rescued the hearing in a mouse model of hereditary deafness. It was a powerful hair cell gene delivery system that could be used for gene therapy of deafness [71].

Oncolytic viruses show unique anti-cancer mechanisms in cancer treatment. Chemotherapeutic drugs combined with oncolytic viruses showed stronger cytotoxicity and oncolytic effects. Someone has studied the systemic delivery of oncolytic adenovirus and paclitaxel encapsulated by EVs. The results have shown that this combination therapy enhanced anticancer effects in lung cancer models both in vitro and in vivo. EVs play a key role in the effective transmission of oncolytic viruses and chemotherapeutic drugs [72].

7. Sources of EVs that can be used for drug delivery

EVs currently used for therapeutic research are mainly derived from the following sources: mesenchymal stem cells (MSCs), dendritic cells (DCs), tumor cells, red blood cells, macrophages and plants. EVs from different sources have different biological characteristics. Materials should be selected according to the purpose of treatment. The characteristics, advantages and disadvantages of EVs from different sources will be described below.

7.1 Mesenchymal stem cells

The MSCs involved in the study of EVs include adipose-derived MSCs, bone marrow MSCs, progenitor cells from different tissues, and so on. MSCs can be extracted from the patient's bone marrow, fat, or other tissues. EVs derived from MSCs are very attractive. Because they have anti-inflammatory, anti-apoptotic and anti-microbial capability, and promote angiogenesis and the repair and regeneration of damaged tissues. As mentioned above, EVs derived from MSCs have been widely used in the treatment of central nervous system diseases, cardiovascular diseases, bone and cartilage damage repair and regeneration, wound repair, and other organ damage repair and regeneration [7–21].

7.2 Dendritic cells

One potential source of therapeutic EVs is immature dendritic cells (imDCs). EVs secreted by imDCs lack surface markers such as CD40, CD86, MHC-I and MHC-II. Therefore, they have low immunogenicity. They can be isolated from CD34+ cells from the patient's peripheral blood. It is one of the preferred sources of therapeutic EVs.

7.3 Tumor cells

The use of EVs derived from tumor cells to deliver drugs and vaccines for immunotherapy is very promising. Tumor EVs can deliver antigens to dendritic cells, thereby inducing T cell-mediated immune responses to tumor cells [73]. As tumor-derived EVs specifically express Tetraspanins, they can target different tissues. This makes it possible to use tumor-derived EVs for tumor-targeting and selective drug delivery [74]. However, tumor-derived EVs also have many potential risks. Due to the presence of Tetraspanins, Urokinase plasminogen activator, Cathepsin D, Vimentin and other molecules derived from the surface of tumor cells [75, 76], they may promote tumor proliferation and metastasis, and Immunosuppressive effect [77–79].

7.4 Red blood cells

Blood EVs mainly secreted by reticulocytes (RTC) are a potential source of safe and sufficient EVs. Because they integrate various membrane proteins including Transferrin (Tf) receptors, but they do not have any immune and cancer stimulating activity [30]. Red blood cell EVs (RBCEV) also have the following advantages: large load; low self-nucleic acid content (red blood cells without nucleus and mitochondria); they can be delivered to a variety of different organs and tissues; large quantities of raw materials and easily available (the raw materials for producing RBCEVs are mainly O-type Blood of blood donors). Using blood EVs as carriers can efficiently target tumors to co-deliver chemotherapeutics and nucleic acid drugs. Significant tumor growth inhibitory effects were observed in tumor-bearing mice. There were no obvious side effects [30].

7.5 Macrophages

Macrophages are an important immune cell in the antigen-presenting cell family. EVs derived from immune cells can mimic immune cells to target tumor cells. Macrophage EVs can transfer miRNAs or proteins to tumor cells, mediate tumor cell resistance to chemotherapy, promote cell invasion and other regulatory effects. Therefore, in the study of tumor treatment of EVs, in addition to using the targeting properties of macrophages-derived EVs, the influence of their contents must also be considered. It has been reported that the contents of EVs derived from macrophages can be removed. Then the EVs were used to carry chemotherapeutic drugs to achieve targeted therapy of triple-negative breast cancer [80].

7.6 Plant-derived EVs

Based on reliable sources and safety, fruits and plants have been used as alternative sources for the isolation of EVs for clinical use [81]. Plant-derived EVs have similar structural characteristics to animal cell-derived EVs. EVs from different plant sources have the physiological functions of the plant from which they are derived. For example, lemon-derived EVs have certain anti-cancer effects. Some researchers have tried to isolate lemon-derived EVs (LDEVs) for the treatment of gastric cancer. LDEVs caused s-phase arrest of gastric cancer cell cycle and induced cell apoptosis. LDEVs could be retained in the organs of the gastrointestinal tract and had strong anti-tumor activity against gastric cancer [82]. The isolated plant EVs can also be used after being engineered. Some researchers isolated EVs from grapefruit, modified the EVs in a targeted manner, and then loaded the anti-tumor drugs doxorubicin and curcumin. These modified EVs could target inflammatory tumors and have anti-inflammatory effects in mouse models [83].

Plant-derived EVs have a wide range of sources, are safe and non-toxic, have low immunogenicity, low cost, and are edible. They have great clinical application potential as edible chemotherapeutic drug carriers.

8. Commercialization progress and potential problems of EVs

8.1 Progress in the commercialization of EVs

So far, no EVs drugs have entered the clinic. Codiak BioSciences, a leading company in the development of engineered EVs as a new type of biopharmaceutical, uses its proprietary engEx platform to engineer EVs with different characteristics, load them with various types of therapeutic molecules and change their orientation, so that they can reach specific cellular targets. Recently, Evox Therapeutics Ltd. and Eli Lilly and Co. reached a cooperation agreement to apply its exosome technology to the system to deliver RNA interference and antisense oligonucleotide drugs to the central nervous system, treating five unspecified Neurological diseases. Carmine Therapeutics is also a gene therapy company based on EVs, established in 2019. Carmine's REGENT technology platform focuses on using red blood cell extracellular vesicles (RBCEV) as drug delivery vehicles. Mantra Bio also joined the emerging group of exosome drug development companies. With the deepening of research, more and more companies will join the field of EVs treatment.

8.2 EVs treatment and COVID-19

The Severe Acute Respiratory Syndrome (which first appeared in December 2019) related to the new coronavirus (COVID-19) has rapidly developed into a pandemic, and the morbidity and mortality rates are increasing worldwide. COVID-19 respiratory tract infection is characterized by an imbalanced immune response, leading to an increased possibility of severe respiratory disease and multiple organ disease.

Because EVs derived from MSCs have anti-inflammatory, anti-apoptotic and anti-microbial capability, promote angiogenesis and the repair and regeneration of damaged tissues. In related lung disease models, including acute lung injury and sepsis, systemic administration of MSC-EVs preparations can modulate immune responses. In a mouse model of pneumonia induced by Escherichia coli, it was found that MSC-EVs administration could enhance the phagocytosis of bacteria. In the pig model, MSC-EVs could reduce influenza virus-induced acute lung injury by inhibiting influenza virus replication. In other disease models, the disease alleviation effect of MSC-EVs on the inflammatory immune response has also been observed. It is speculated that they may also have anti-COVID-19 efficacy. In cell therapy research for COVID-19, some registered clinical trials have turned their targets to EVs in the conditioned medium of MSCs. MSC-EVs can be administered intravenously (ChiCTR2000030484) or by inhalation (NCT04276987, ChiCTR2000030261).

However, before using MSC-EVs for COVID-19 patients, many other issues should be considered, such as the huge heterogeneity of MSC-EVs composition and source. In fact, comparing MSC-EVs harvested from the conditioned medium of bone marrow MSCs derived from different donors, there are significant differences in cytokine content and different therapeutic effects. In addition to immune regulation, MSC-EVs can also control other biological processes and may cause unpredictable side effects. For example, increasing the risk of thrombosis.

In short, in order to reduce the risk of potential life-threatening side effects, International Society for Extracellular Vesicles (ISEV) and International Society for Cell and Gene Therapy (ISCT) strongly require that the clinical data from reasonable clinical trial should be carefully weighed. The EV preparations with good characteristics and produced under strict GMP conditions and appropriate regulatory supervision could be used. Any application of EVs should be carefully evaluated [84].

8.3 Potential problems in the industrialization of EVs

The potential application of EVs in new diagnostic and therapeutic strategies has attracted increasing attention. However, due to the inherent complex biogenesis of EVs and their huge heterogeneity in size, composition and source, the research of

EVs still faces huge challenges. It is necessary to establish a standardized method to solve the heterogeneity of EVs and the analysis of pre-processing and analysis of sources of variability in the study of EVs. The quality standards, extraction specifications and especially the stability of preparation conditions for therapeutic EVs also need to be clarified.

In addition, the diversity and uncertainty of EVs content are also issues that need to be considered in the application. Before metastasis, malignant tumor cells use EVs to modify the microenvironment of the organ targeted by cancer metastasis, making it a suitable "soil" for tumor cell growth. The contents of EVs secreted by most tumor cells play a role in promoting tumor metastasis and progression. As mentioned earlier in this article, macrophage EVs can transfer miRNAs and proteins to tumor cells, mediate tumor cell resistance to chemotherapy, promote cell invasion and other regulatory effects. Therefore, if EVs from such sources are used as drug carriers, it is particularly important to first remove the adverse effects of their contents.

9. Conclusion

As an important medium of intercellular communication, EVs play an important physiological function and are also involved in the occurrence and development of a variety of diseases. In recent years, there have been numerous studies on the treatment of related diseases with EVs from different cell sources, and EV has shown its unique advantages in drug transportation. EVs are similar to natural liposomes, which can enhance the function of EVs to treat specific diseases through targeting modification and delivery of functional active substances and other technical modifications according to the characteristics of different diseases. EVs with improved function have shown obvious advantages in the treatment of tumors and difficult diseases of central nervous system. However, the clinical application of EVs technology is still in its infancy, and the challenges it faces are accompanied by the possibility of numerous new discoveries and new technologies. We expect that with the continuous in-depth research, EVs as a new drug carrier in the treatment of a variety of diseases will bring more and greater surprises.

Acknowledgements

This work was supported by the National Key R&D Program of China (2018YFA0900900), and the National Natural Science Foundation of China (81773251 and 81702735).

Author details

Chunying Liu, Xuejing Lin and Changqing Su*
Department of Molecular Oncology, National Center for Liver Cancer, Eastern Hepatobiliary Surgery Hospital, Second Military Medical University, Shanghai, China

*Address all correspondence to: suchangqing@gmail.com

References

[1] Gurunathan S, Kang MH, Jeyaraj M, Qasim M, Kim JH. Review of the isolation, characterization, biological function, and multifarious therapeutic approaches of exosomes. Cells. 2019;8:307. DOI: 10.3390/cells8040307

[2] Shao H, Im H, Castro CM, Breakefield X, Weissleder R, Lee H. New technologies for analysis of extracellular vesicles. Chem Rev. 2018;118:1917-50. DOI: 10.1021/acs.chemrev.7b00534

[3] Théry C, Zitvogel L, Amigorena S. Exosomes: composition, biogenesis and function. Nat Rev Immunol. 2002;2:569-79. DOI: 10.1038/nri855

[4] Colombo M, Raposo G, Théry C. Biogenesis, secretion, and intercellular interactions of exosomes and other extracellular vesicles. Annu Rev Cell Dev Biol. 2014;30:255-89. DOI: 10.1146/annurev-cellbio-101512-122326

[5] van Niel G, D'Angelo G, Raposo G. Shedding light on the cell biology of extracellular vesicles. Nat Rev Mol Cell Biol. 2018;19:213-28. DOI: 10.1038/nrm.2017.125

[6] Kamerkar S, LeBleu VS, Sugimoto H, Yang S, Ruivo CF, Melo SA, et al. Exosomes facilitate therapeutic targeting of oncogenic KRAS in pancreatic cancer. Nature. 2017;546: 498-503. DOI: 10.1038/nature22341

[7] Li L, Zhang Y, Mu J, Chen J, Zhang C, Cao H, et al. Transplantation of human mesenchymal stem cell-derived exosomes immobilized in an adhesive hydrogel for effective treatment of spinal cord injury. Nano Lett. 2020;20:4298-305. DOI: 10.1021/acs.nanolett.0c00929

[8] Hu G, Xia Y, Zhang J, Chen Y, Yuan J, Niu X, et al. ESC-sEVs rejuvenate senescent hippocampal NSCs by activating lysosomes to improve cognitive dysfunction in vascular dementia. Adv Sci (Weinh). 2020;7:1903330. DOI: 10.1002/advs.201903330

[9] Wu Q, Wang J, Tan WLW, Jiang Y, Wang S, Li Q, et al. Extracellular vesicles from human embryonic stem cell-derived cardiovascular progenitor cells promote cardiac infarct healing through reducing cardiomyocyte death and promoting angiogenesis. Cell Death Dis. 2020;11:354. DOI: 10.1038/s41419-020-2508-y

[10] Khan M, Nickoloff E, Abramova T, Johnson J, Verma SK, Krishnamurthy P, et al. Embryonic stem cell-derived exosomes promote endogenous repair mechanisms and enhance cardiac function following myocardial infarction. Circulation research. 2015;117:52-64. DOI: 10.1161/CIRCRESAHA.117.305990

[11] Wang Y, Zhang L, Li Y, Chen L, Wang X, Guo W, et al. Exosomes/microvesicles from induced pluripotent stem cells deliver cardioprotective miRNAs and prevent cardiomyocyte apoptosis in the ischemic myocardium. International journal of cardiology. 2015;192:61-9. DOI: 10.1016/j.ijcard.2015.05.020

[12] Bouchareychas L, Duong P, Covarrubias S, Alsop E, Phu TA, Chung A, et al. Macrophage exosomes resolve atherosclerosis by regulating hematopoiesis and inflammation via microRNA cargo. Cell Rep. 2020;32:107881. DOI: 10.1016/j.celrep.2020.107881

[13] Lei X, He N, Zhu L, Zhou M, Zhang K, Wang C, et al. Mesenchymal stem cell-derived extracellular vesicles attenuate radiation-induced lung injury via miRNA-214-3p. Antioxid Redox Signal. 2020. DOI: 10.1089/ars.2019.7965

[14] Hu S, Li Z, Lutz H, Huang K, Su T, Cores J, et al. Dermal exosomes containing miR-218-5p promote hair regeneration by regulating β-catenin signaling. Sci Adv. 2020;6:eaba1685. DOI: 10.1126/sciadv.aba1685

[15] Yan B, Zhang Y, Liang C, Liu B, Ding F, Wang Y, et al. Stem cell-derived exosomes prevent pyroptosis and repair ischemic muscle injury through a novel exosome/circHIPK3/ FOXO3a pathway. Theranostics. 2020;10:6728-42. DOI: 10.7150/thno.42259

[16] Zhang S, Yang Y, Jia S, Chen H, Duan Y, Li X, et al. Exosome-like vesicles derived from Hertwig's epithelial root sheath cells promote the regeneration of dentin-pulp tissue. Theranostics. 2020;10:5914-31. DOI: 10.7150/thno.43156

[17] Bian B, Zhao C, He X, Gong Y, Ren C, Ge L, et al. Exosomes derived from neural progenitor cells preserve photoreceptors during retinal degeneration by inactivating microglia. J Extracell Vesicles. 2020;9:1748931. DOI: 10.1080/20013078.2020.1748931

[18] Fafián-Labora JA, Rodríguez-Navarro JA, O'Loghlen A. Small extracellular vesicles have GST activity and ameliorate senescence-related tissue damage. Cell Metab. 2020;32:71-86 e5. DOI: 10.1016/j.cmet.2020.06.004

[19] Li CJ, Fang QH, Liu ML, Lin JN. Current understanding of the role of Adipose-derived Extracellular Vesicles in Metabolic Homeostasis and Diseases: Communication from the distance between cells/tissues. Theranostics. 2020;10:7422-35. DOI: 10.7150/thno.42167

[20] Zhang H, Wang J, Ren T, Huang Y, Liang X, Yu Y, et al. Bone marrow mesenchymal stem cell-derived exosomal miR-206 inhibits osteosarcoma progression by targeting TRA2B. Cancer Lett. 2020;490:54-65. DOI: 10.1016/j.canlet.2020.07.008

[21] He Z, Li W, Zheng T, Liu D, Zhao S. Human umbilical cord mesenchymal stem cells-derived exosomes deliver microRNA-375 to downregulate ENAH and thus retard esophageal squamous cell carcinoma progression. J Exp Clin Cancer Res. 2020;39:140. DOI: 10.1186/s13046-020-01631-w

[22] Gazdic M, Volarevic V, Harrell CR, Fellabaum C, Jovicic N, Arsenijevic N, et al. Stem cells therapy for spinal cord injury. Int J Mol Sci. 2018 Mar 30;19:1039. DOI: 10.3390/ijms19041039

[23] González C, Bonilla S, Flores AI, Cano E, Liste I. An update on human stem cell-based therapy in Parkinson's disease. Curr Stem Cell Res Ther. 2016;11:561-8. DOI: 10.2174/1574888x10666150531172612

[24] Tang W. Challenges and advances in stem cell therapy. Biosci Trends. 2019;13:286. DOI: 10.5582/bst.2019.01241

[25] Isomi M, Sadahiro T, Ieda M. Progress and challenge of cardiac regeneration to treat heart failure. J Cardiol. 2019;73:97-101. DOI: 10.1016/j.jjcc.2018.10.002

[26] Adamiak M, Cheng G, Bobis-Wozowicz S, Zhao L, Kedracka-Krok S, Samanta A, et al. Induced pluripotent stem cell (iPSC)-derived extracellular vesicles are safer and more effective for cardiac repair than iPSCs. Circ Res. 2018;122:296-309. DOI: 10.1161/CIRCRESAHA.117.311769

[27] Dougherty JA, Kumar N, Noor M, Angelos MG, Khan M, Chen CA. Extracellular vesicles released by human induced-pluripotent stem cell-derived cardiomyocytes promote angiogenesis. Front Physiol. 2018;9:1794. DOI: 10.3389/fphys.2018.01794

[28] Kato T, Fahrmann JF, Hanash SM, Vykoukal J. Extracellular vesicles mediate B cell immune response and

are a potential target for cancer therapy. Cells. 2020;9:1518. DOI: 10.3390/cells9061518

[29] Usman WM, Pham TC, Kwok YY, Vu LT, Ma V, Peng B, et al. Efficient RNA drug delivery using red blood cell extracellular vesicles. Nat Commun. 2018;9:2359. DOI: 10.1038/s41467-018-04791-8

[30] Zhan Q, Yi K, Qi H, Li S, Li X, Wang Q, et al. Engineering blood exosomes for tumor-targeting efficient gene/chemo combination therapy. Theranostics. 2020;10:7889-905. DOI: 10.7150/thno.45028

[31] Xu Q, Zhang Z, Zhao L, Qin Y, Cai H, Geng Z, et al. Tropism-facilitated delivery of CRISPR/Cas9 system with chimeric antigen receptor-extracellular vesicles against B-cell malignancies. J Control Release. 2020;326:455-67. DOI: 10.1016/j.jconrel.2020.07.033

[32] Yang L, Han B, Zhang Z, Wang S, Bai Y, Zhang Y, et al. Extracellular vesicle-mediated delivery of circular RNA SCMH1 promotes functional recovery in rodent and nonhuman primate ischemic stroke models. Circulation. 2020;142:556-74. DOI: 10.1161/CIRCULATIONAHA.120.045765

[33] Wang X, Zhang H, Bai M, Ning T, Ge S, Deng T, et al. Exosomes serve as nanoparticles to deliver anti-miR-214 to reverse chemoresistance to cisplatin in gastric cancer. Mol Ther. 2018;26:774-83. DOI: 10.1016/j.ymthe.2018.01.001

[34] Yang T, Fogarty B, LaForge B, Aziz S, Pham T, Lai L, et al. Delivery of small interfering RNA to inhibit vascular endothelial growth factor in zebrafish using natural brain endothelia cell-secreted exosome nanovesicles for the treatment of brain cancer. AAPS J. 2016;19:475-86. DOI: 10.1208/s12248-016-0015-y

[35] Alvarez-Erviti L, Seow Y, Yin H, Betts C, Lakhal S, Wood MJ. Delivery of siRNA to the mouse brain by systemic injection of targeted exosomes. Nat Biotechnol. 2011;29:341-5. DOI: 10.1038/nbt.1807

[36] Luo Q, Guo D, Liu G, Chen G, Hang M, Jin M. Exosomes from miR-126-overexpressing Adscs are therapeutic in relieving acute myocardial ischaemic injury. Cell Physiol Biochem. 2017;44:2105-16. DOI: 10.1159/000485949

[37] Zhang H, Wang Y, Bai M, Wang J, Zhu K, Liu R, et al. Exosomes serve as nanoparticles to suppress tumor growth and angiogenesis in gastric cancer by delivering hepatocyte growth factor siRNA. Cancer Sci. 2017;109:629-41. DOI: 10.1111/cas.13488

[38] Kojima R, Bojar D, Rizzi G, Hamri GC, El-Baba MD, Saxena P, et al. Designer exosomes produced by implanted cells intracerebrally deliver therapeutic cargo for Parkinson's disease treatment. Nat Commun. 2018;9:1305. DOI: 10.1038/s41467-018-03733-8

[39] Batagov AO, Kuznetsov VA, Kurochkin IV. Identification of nucleotide patterns enriched in secreted RNAs as putative cis-acting elements targeting them to exosome nano-vesicles. BMC Genomics. 2011;12 Suppl 3(Suppl 3):S18. DOI: 10.1186/1471-2164-12-S3-S18

[40] Ausländer S, Ausländer D, Müller M, Wieland M, Fussenegger M. Programmable single-cell mammalian biocomputers. Nature. 2012;487:123-7. DOI: 10.1038/nature11149

[41] Saito H, Fujita Y, Kashida S, Hayashi K, Inoue T. Synthetic human cell fate regulation by protein-driven RNA switches. Nat Commun. 2011;2:160. DOI: 10.1038/ncomms1157

[42] Saito H, Kobayashi T, Hara T, Fujita Y, Hayashi K, Furushima R, et al. Synthetic translational regulation by

an L7Ae-kink-turn RNP switch. Nat Chem Biol. 2010;6:71-8. DOI: 10.1038/nchembio.273

[43] Ke C, Hou H, Li J, Su K, Huang C, Lin Y, et al. Extracellular vesicle delivery of TRAIL eradicates resistant tumor growth in combination with CDK inhibition by Dinaciclib. Cancers (Basel). 2020;12:1157. DOI: 10.3390/cancers12051157

[44] Xu Z, Tsai HI, Xiao Y, Wu Y, Su D, Yang M, et al. Engineering programmed death ligand-1/cytotoxic T-lymphocyte-associated antigen-4 dual-targeting nanovesicles for immunosuppressive therapy in transplantation. ACS Nano. 2020;14:7959-69. DOI: 10.1021/acsnano.9b09065

[45] Gee P, Lung MSY, Okuzaki Y, Sasakawa N, Iguchi T, Makita Y, et al. Extracellular nanovesicles for packaging of CRISPR-Cas9 protein and sgRNA to induce therapeutic exon skipping. Nat Commun. 2020;11:1334. DOI: 10.1038/s41467-020-14957-y

[46] Haney MJ, Klyachko NL, Zhao Y, Gupta R, Plotnikova EG, He Z, et al. Exosomes as drug delivery vehicles for Parkinson's disease therapy. J Control Release. 2015;207:18-30. DOI: 10.1016/j.jconrel.2015.03.033

[47] Yang J, Wu S, Hou L, Zhu D, Yin S, Yang G, et al. Therapeutic effects of simultaneous delivery of nerve growth factor mRNA and protein via exosomes on cerebral ischemia. Mol Ther Nucleic Acids. 2020;21:512-22. DOI: 10.1016/j.omtn.2020.06.013

[48] Hoshino A, Costa-Silva B, Shen TL, Rodrigues G, Hashimoto A, Tesic Mark M, et al. Tumour exosome integrins determine organotropic metastasis. Nature. 2015;527:329-35. DOI: 10.1038/nature15756

[49] Rak J. Cancer: Organ-seeking vesicles. Nature. 2015;527:312-4. DOI: 10.1038/nature15642

[50] Tian Y, Li S, Song J, Ji T, Zhu M, Anderson GJ, et al. A doxorubicin delivery platform using engineered natural membrane vesicle exosomes for targeted tumor therapy. Biomaterials. 2014;35:2383-90. DOI: 10.1016/j.biomaterials.2013.11.083

[51] Yang J, Zhang X, Chen X, Wang L, Yang G. Exosome mediated delivery of miR-124 promotes neurogenesis after ischemia. Mol Ther Nucleic Acids. 2017;7:278-87. DOI: 10.1016/j.omtn.2017.04.010

[52] Chen W, Yang M, Bai J, Li X, Kong X, Gao Y, et al. Exosome-modified tissue engineered blood vessel for endothelial progenitor cell capture and targeted siRNA delivery. Macromol Biosci. 2018;18. DOI: 10.1002/mabi.201700242

[53] Liu C, Su C. Design strategies and application progress of therapeutic exosomes. Theranostics. 2019;9:1015-28. DOI: 10.7150/thno.30853

[54] Hall J, Prabhakar S, Balaj L, Lai CP, Cerione RA, Breakefield XO. Delivery of therapeutic proteins via extracellular vesicles: Review and potential treatments for Parkinson's disease, glioma, and schwannoma. Cell Mol Neurobiol. 2016;36:417-27. DOI: 10.1007/s10571-015-0309-0

[55] Di Bonito P, Chiozzini C, Arenaccio C, Anticoli S, Manfredi F, Olivetta E, et al. Antitumor HPV E7-specific CTL activity elicited by in vivo engineered exosomes produced through DNA inoculation. Int J Nanomedicine. 2017;12:4579-91. DOI: 10.2147/IJN.S131309

[56] Meyer C, Losacco J, Stickney Z, Li L, Marriott G, Lu B. Pseudotyping exosomes for enhanced protein delivery in mammalian cells. Int J Nanomedicine. 2017;12:3153-70. DOI: 10.2147/IJN.S133430

[57] Zheng P, Luo Q, Wang W, Li J, Wang T, Wang P, et al. Tumor-associated

macrophages-derived exosomes promote the migration of gastric cancer cells by transfer of functional Apolipoprotein E. Cell Death Dis. 2018;9:434. DOI: 10.1038/s41419-018-0465-5

[58] Simpson RJ, Jensen SS, Lim JW. Proteomic profiling of exosomes: current perspectives. Proteomics. 2008;8:4083-99. DOI: 10.1002/pmic.200800109

[59] Yim N, Ryu SW, Choi K, Lee KR, Lee S, Choi H, et al. Exosome engineering for efficient intracellular delivery of soluble proteins using optically reversible protein-protein interaction module. Nat Commun. 2016;7:12277. DOI: 10.1038/ncomms12277

[60] Cheng Y, Schorey JS. Targeting soluble proteins to exosomes using a ubiquitin tag. Biotechnol Bioeng. 2015;113:1315-24. DOI: 10.1002/bit.25884

[61] Shen B, Wu N, Yang JM, Gould SJ. Protein targeting to exosomes/microvesicles by plasma membrane anchors. J Biol Chem. 2011;286:14383-95. DOI: 10.1074/jbc.M110.208660

[62] Wan Y, Wang L, Zhu C, Zheng Q, Wang G, Tong J, et al. Aptamer-conjugated extracellular nanovesicles for targeted drug delivery. Cancer Res. 2018;78:798-808. DOI: 10.1158/0008-5472.CAN-17-2880

[63] Zhang D, Qin X, Wu T, Qiao Q, Song Q, Zhang Z. Extracellular vesicles based self-grown gold nanopopcorn for combinatorial chemo-photothermal therapy. Biomaterials. 2019;197:220-8. DOI: 10.1016/j.biomaterials.2019.01.024

[64] Zarovni N, Corrado A, Guazzi P, Zocco D, Lari E, Radano G, et al. Integrated isolation and quantitative analysis of exosome shuttled proteins and nucleic acids using immunocapture approaches. Methods. 2015;87:46-58. DOI: 10.1016/j.ymeth.2015.05.028

[65] Kim MS, Haney MJ, Zhao Y, Mahajan V, Deygen I, Klyachko NL, et al. Development of exosome-encapsulated paclitaxel to overcome MDR in cancer cells. Nanomedicine. 2015;12:655-64. DOI: 10.1016/j.nano.2015.10.012

[66] Pascucci L, Coccè V, Bonomi A, Ami D, Ceccarelli P, Ciusani E, et al. Paclitaxel is incorporated by mesenchymal stromal cells and released in exosomes that inhibit in vitro tumor growth: a new approach for drug delivery. J Control Release. 2014;192:262-70. DOI: 10.1016/j.jconrel.2014.07.042

[67] Gao Y, Zhang H, Zhou N, Xu P, Wang J, Jin X, et al. Methotrexate-loaded tumour-cell-derived microvesicles can relieve biliary obstruction in patients with extrahepatic cholangiocarcinoma. Nat Biomed Eng. 2020;4:743-53. DOI: 10.1038/s41551-020-0583-0

[68] Hudry E, Martin C, Gandhi S, György B, Scheffer DI, Mu D, et al. Exosome-associated AAV vector as a robust and convenient neuroscience tool. Gene Ther. 2016;23:380-92. DOI: 10.1038/gt.2016.11

[69] György B, Fitzpatrick Z, Crommentuijn MH, Mu D, Maguire CA. Naturally enveloped AAV vectors for shielding neutralizing antibodies and robust gene delivery in vivo. Biomaterials. 2014;35:7598-609. DOI: 10.1016/j.biomaterials.2014.05.032

[70] Wassmer SJ, Carvalho LS, György B, Vandenberghe LH, Maguire CA. Exosome-associated AAV2 vector mediates robust gene delivery into the murine retina upon intravitreal injection. Sci Rep. 2017;7:45329. DOI: 10.1038/srep45329

[71] György B, Sage C, Indzhykulian AA, Scheffer DI, Brisson AR, Tan S, et al. Rescue of hearing by gene delivery to inner-ear hair cells using

exosome-associated AAV. Mol Ther. 2017;25:379-91. DOI: 10.1016/j.ymthe.2016.12.010

[72] Garofalo M, Saari H, Somersalo P, Crescenti D, Kuryk L, Aksela L, et al. Antitumor effect of oncolytic virus and paclitaxel encapsulated in extracellular vesicles for lung cancer treatment. J Control Release. 2018;283:223-34. DOI: 10.1016/j.jconrel.2018.05.015

[73] Wolfers J, Lozier A, Raposo G, Regnault A, Théry C, Masurier C, et al. Tumor-derived exosomes are a source of shared tumor rejection antigens for CTL cross-priming. Nat Med. 2001;7:297-303. DOI: 10.1038/85438

[74] Rana S, Yue S, Stadel D, Zöller M. Toward tailored exosomes: the exosomal tetraspanin web contributes to target cell selection. Int J Biochem Cell Biol. 2012;44:1574-84. DOI: 10.1016/j.biocel.2012.06.018

[75] Zomer A, Maynard C, Verweij FJ, Kamermans A, Schäfer R, Beerling E, et al. In vivo imaging reveals extracellular vesicle-mediated phenocopying of metastatic behavior. Cell. 2015;161:1046-57. DOI: 10.1016/j.cell.2015.04.042

[76] Harris DA, Patel SH, Gucek M, Hendrix A, Westbroek W, Taraska JW. Exosomes released from breast cancer carcinomas stimulate cell movement. PLoS One. 2015;10:e0117495. DOI: 10.1371/journal.pone.0117495

[77] Tomihari M, Chung JS, Akiyoshi H, Cruz PD, Jr., Ariizumi K. DC-HIL/glycoprotein Nmb promotes growth of melanoma in mice by inhibiting the activation of tumor-reactive T cells. Cancer Res. 2010;70:5778-87. DOI: 10.1158/0008-5472.CAN-09-2538

[78] Kim JW, Wieckowski E, Taylor DD, Reichert TE, Watkins S, Whiteside TL. Fas ligand-positive membranous vesicles isolated from sera of patients with oral cancer induce apoptosis of activated T lymphocytes. Clin Cancer Res. 2005;11:1010-20.

[79] Luan X, Sansanaphongpricha K, Myers I, Chen H, Yuan H, Sun D. Engineering exosomes as refined biological nanoplatforms for drug delivery. Acta Pharmacol Sin. 2017;38:754-63. DOI: 10.1038/aps.2017.12

[80] Li S, Wu Y, Ding F, Yang J, Li J, Gao X, et al. Engineering macrophage-derived exosomes for targeted chemotherapy of triple-negative breast cancer. Nanoscale. 2020;12:10854-62. DOI: 10.1039/d0nr00523a

[81] Ju S, Mu J, Dokland T, Zhuang X, Wang Q, Jiang H, et al. Grape exosome-like nanoparticles induce intestinal stem cells and protect mice from DSS-induced colitis. Mol Ther. 2013;21:1345-57. DOI: 10.1038/mt.2013.64

[82] Yang M, Liu X, Luo Q, Xu L, Chen F. An efficient method to isolate lemon derived extracellular vesicles for gastric cancer therapy. J Nanobiotechnology. 2020;18:100. DOI: 10.1186/s12951-020-00656-9

[83] Wang Q, Ren Y, Mu J, Egilmez NK, Zhuang X, Deng Z, et al. Grapefruit-derived nanovectors use an activated leukocyte trafficking pathway to deliver therapeutic agents to inflammatory tumor sites. Cancer Res. 2015;75:2520-9. DOI: 10.1158/0008-5472.CAN-14-3095

[84] Börger V, Weiss DJ, Anderson JD, Borràs FE, Bussolati B, Carter DRF, et al. International Society for Extracellular Vesicles and International Society for Cell and Gene Therapy statement on extracellular vesicles from mesenchymal stromal cells and other cells: considerations for potential therapeutic agents to suppress coronavirus disease-19. Cytotherapy. 2020;22:482-5. DOI: 10.1016/j.jcyt.2020.05.002

Section 3

Theranostics with Nanomaterials

Chapter 5

Graphene-Based Nanosystems: Versatile Nanotools for Theranostics and Bioremediation

Marlene Lúcio, Eduarda Fernandes, Hugo Gonçalves, Sofia Machado, Andreia C. Gomes and Maria Elisabete C.D. Real Oliveira

Abstract

Since its revolutionary discovery in 2004, graphene— a two-dimensional (2D) nanomaterial consisting of single-layer carbon atoms packed in a honeycomb lattice — was thoroughly discussed for a broad variety of applications including quantum physics, nanoelectronics, energy efficiency, and catalysis. Graphene and graphene-based nanomaterials (GBNs) have also captivated the interest of researchers for innovative biomedical applications since the first publication on the use of graphene as a nanocarrier for the delivery of anticancer drugs in 2008. Today, GBNs have evolved into hybrid combinations of graphene and other elements (e.g., drugs or other bioactive compounds, polymers, lipids, and nanoparticles). In the context of developing theranostic (therapeutic + diagnostic) tools, which combine multiple therapies with imaging strategies to track the distribution of therapeutic agents in the body, the multipurpose character of the GBNs hybrid systems has been further explored. Because each therapy and imaging strategy has inherent advantages and disadvantages, a mixture of complementary strategies is interesting as it will result in a synergistic theranostic effect. The flexibility of GBNs cannot be limited to their biomedical applications and, these nanosystems emerge as a viable choice for an indirect effect on health by their future use as environmental cleaners. Indeed, GBNs can be used in bioremediation approaches alone or combined with other techniques such as phytoremediation. In summary, without ignoring the difficulties that GBNs still present before being deemed translatable to clinical and environmental applications, the purpose of this chapter is to provide an overview of the remarkable potential of GBNs on health by presenting examples of their versatility as nanotools for theranostics and bioremediation.

Keywords: Graphene-based nanomaterials, graphene, graphene oxide, reduced graphene oxide, graphene quantum dots, cancer theranostics, green synthesis, bioremediation

1. Introduction

Since its first serendipitous but groundbreaking discovery by Geim and Novoselov in 2004 [1], followed by the 2010 Nobel Prize in Physics, graphene has drawn tremendous interest from scientists from every direction to exploit many of its special features. Indeed, graphene and graphene-based nanomaterials (GBNs) have distinctive mechanical, electronic, optical, and chemical properties [2–4]. Graphene and GBNs can therefore be found in numerous applications in the areas of electronics, physics, and material science [5–7]. In recent times, considering an emerging opinion on the eco-friendly characteristics of graphene and its derivatives, researchers have agreed to use these nanomaterials in other fields of science, for example in medical [8–13] and environmental applications in bioremediation [14–21].

One of the most interesting applications of GBNs in the medicine field is its use as theranostic tools, i.e. taking advantage of its properties to provide a combination strategy for both therapy and diagnosis [8]. Multiple combinations of different therapeutic and diagnostic strategies are currently being used to achieve a therapeutic effect with GBNs. Since each strategy has inherent advantages and limitations, a combination of complementary strategies can result in a synergistic theranostic effect [8]. Of all diseases, the synergistic theranostic effects of GBNs can be more significant in cancer. In fact, despite all the resources expended in clinical advances, cancer remains the world's leading cause of death, with a confirmed mortality rate of 8.8 million by 2015. In addition, the World Health Organization (WHO) and International Agency for Research on Cancer (IARC) expect all cases of cancer to rise to 21.2 million by 2030 [22, 23]. With conventional approaches to cancer treatment, such as chemotherapy and radiation, tumor-initiating cells also designated as cancer stem cells (CSCs), are hard to eradicate [24]. The survival of residual CSCs is therefore believed to drive the onset of tumor recurrence, distant metastasis, and drug resistance, which is a major clinical problem for effective cancer treatment [24]. Therefore, new cancer therapy approaches such as GBNs are urgently necessary to address this clinical need [8, 24].

Another field that requires investment in research is the use of GBNs in bioremediation. Air, water, and soil pollution is a worldwide challenge for the environment and human society [17, 18, 25]. The removal from the environment of multiple pollutants, including inorganic and organic compounds, is a growing concern [17, 18, 25]. The most harmful and hazardous pollutants that have been the focus of the GBNs' bioremediation research will be discussed in this chapter and listed according to the following classes: volatile organic compounds, inorganic metals, organic dyes, polycyclic aromatic hydrocarbons, pharmaceuticals, pesticides. In water sources and the atmosphere, these chemical pollutants also have the property of degrading and producing carcinogenic and mutagenic compounds [20]. In addition, microbial drug resistance can also be caused by bioaccumulation of contaminants such as pharmaceutical drugs, pesticides and their by-products in water bodies [20]. Therefore, pollution damages ecosystems but also affects human health, and the large number of pollutants emitted annually by industries and households have had a major impact on the environment and human existence.

This chapter presents an overview of the properties of graphene and GBNs and their synthesis by classical and green methods. In addition, the use of GBNs will be described either in medicine (as theranostic tools) or in bioremediation (as adsorbents and photocatalysts) and these different aspects will be presented as part of their versatile beneficial use when applied to human health.

2. Graphene and GBNs

Graphene is a single layer of sp^2 hybridized carbon atoms bound together in a planar 2D honeycomb structure.

GBNs are graphene-like structures that can be obtained from graphene or graphite as the starting material, but that possess sp^2 and sp^3 hybridized carbon atoms and differ from one another in terms of surface chemistry, number of defects and lateral dimensions (**Table 1**). GBNs include graphene derivatives, such as graphene oxide (GO), reduced graphene oxide (rGO), graphene quantum dots (GQDs). GO is a highly oxidized form of graphene that contains oxygen functional groups (e.g., epoxide –O–; carboxyl –COOH; hydroxyl –OH) either in the plane or at the edges. rGO is a reduced form of GO where most of its functional oxygen groups have been removed. As a result of oxygen removal processes, rGO has more in-plane defects than GO and graphene. On the other hand, due to oxidation processes, GO has more defects than pristine graphene. GQDs consist of one or more layers (up to ten layers) of graphene or rGOs with a lateral size below 30 nm.

3. Properties of graphene and GBNs

Many fascinating properties of graphene, including strong thermal and electrical conductivity, large surface area and excellent mechanical properties, have been discovered since 2004 (**Table 1**). Further data on the properties of graphene can be found elsewhere [37, 38]. Herein, we focused on the properties of graphene and GBNs that are most significant for their biomedical and environmental applications and emphasized how these exceptional properties are connected to the special 2D carbon atomic honeycomb structure of graphene and its derivatives.

3.1 Mechanical properties

Because of the 2D carbon atomic honeycomb arrangement, each carbon atom is covalently bound to three neighbouring atoms inside a graphene layer. The tight C-C covalent bonds are responsible for graphene's extraordinary structural rigidity and a single defect-free graphene sheet is thus approximately 200 times mechanically stronger than steel. This explains the outstanding mechanical parameters of graphene: Young's modulus of 1 TPa, Poisson's ratio of 0.149 GPa and fracture strength of 130 GPa [27] (**Table 1**).

The mechanical properties of GO and rGO are significantly affected compared to graphene and depend on the surface groups and defects left over from oxidation or other treatment processes. However, the rigidity of these GBNs is still particularly high. Graphene's extraordinary structural rigidity and the still excellent mechanical properties of GBNs mean that these nanomaterials can potentially be used in medical devices, hydrogels, biodegradable films, electrospun fibres and other tissue engineering scaffolds to fill or strengthen the structures of these materials [39].

3.2 Thermal and electrical properties

Graphene is a monoatomic layer of sp^2 hybridized carbon atoms arranged as a honeycomb lattice. The π–π bonds below and above the carbon atomic plane impart exceptional thermal and electrical conductivity to graphene. In fact, a carbon atom normally has four electrons for bonding, but in graphene every atom allocates a single unbound electron that walks freely through the crystal lattice and leads to excellent electrical and thermal conductivity [28]. Defect-free graphene has therefore been reported to have a thermal conductivity between 4500 and 5200 W/m·K [28]. Additionally, graphene exhibits an ultra-high electron mobility (25×10^4 cm^2/V·s) and an electrical conductivity of 10^4 S/cm [29] (**Table 1**).

Graphene or GBNs	Structure and physicochemical properties	Mechanical Properties	Electrical and thermal Properties	Optical properties
Graphene	• Monoatomic layer of sp^2 hybridized carbon atoms arranged as a honeycomb lattice • Hydrophobic • Establishes π-π stacking and hydrophobic interactions [26] 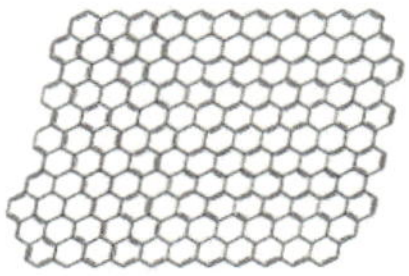	• E = 1000 GPa • FS = 130 GPa [27]	• $\sigma = 10^4$ S/cm • κ = 5000 W/m·K [28, 29]	• 97.7% optical transmittance • NIR absorption [30]
GO	• Sp^3 and sp^2 domains with oxygen functional groups • Amphiphilic • Establishes π-π stacking, H bonds, electrostatic and hydrophobic interactions [31] 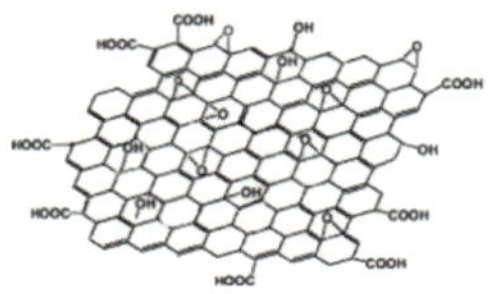	• E = 220 GPa • FS = 120 GPa [32, 33]	• $\sigma = 10^{-1}$ S/cm • κ = 0.5–1 W/m·K [29, 34]	• Intrinsic photoluminescence with UV excitation and tuneable emission in UV–Vis range • NIR absorption [31]
rGO	• Sp^3 and larger sp^2 domains than GO with less hydrophilic groups • Hydrophobic (less than graphene and more than GO) • Establishes π-π stacking, and hydrophobic interactions [31] 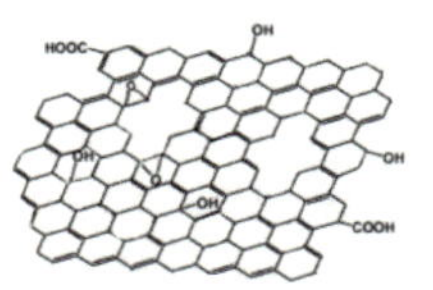	• E = 250 GPa • FS n/a [32]	• $\sigma = 2 \times 10^2$ S/cm • κ = 3–51 W/m·K [34, 35]	• 60–90% optical transmittance • Strong photoluminescence quenching effect [31] • Enhanced NIR absorption (6 times higher than GO) [36]
GQDs	• Small sp^3 and sp^2 domains with oxygen functional groups • Amphiphilic • Establishes π-π stacking, H bonds, electrostatic and hydrophobic interactions [31] 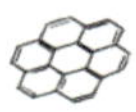	• n/a	• n/a	• Intrinsic photoluminescence with UV excitation and tuneable emission in UV–Vis range • NIR absorption [31]

Abbreviations and symbols: GBNs – Graphene based nanomaterials; GO – Graphene oxide; rGO – Reduced graphene oxide; GQDs – Graphene quantum dots; n/a – not available; NIR –near infrared; E – *Young's modulus;* FS – *Fracture strength;* κ – *Thermal conductivity;* σ – *Electrical conductivity.*

Table 1.
Summary of the properties of the family of graphene nanomaterials.

Defects caused by GO and rGO manufacturing lead to disruption of graphene sp^2 bonding orbitals and the addition of abundant surface groups that impede electron and heat flow, thereby reducing electronic and thermal conductivity of these GBNs [10, 40]. However, the electrical conductivity can be greatly improved upon GO reduction and conversion into rGO, although it is always smaller than that of graphene, as even after reduction, the rGO contains residual sp^3 bonded carbon to oxygen, which interferes with the electron movement through the rest of the sp^2 clusters [10, 40, 41].

As a result of its superior electrical conductivity and thermal properties, graphene is the nanomaterial of choice for electronic applications, but also for biomedical applications for cell potential assessment and as a substrate for biosensors and conductive cell culture devices [42–45].

3.3 Physicochemical properties

The first special physicochemical characteristics of graphene are its high surface area combined with the sp^2 network (**Table 1**). These two characteristics confer great reactivity to graphene. The graphene planar and electron networks can engage in various electrophilic replacement reactions such as click reactions, cyclo-additions, and reactions to carbine insertion. Moreover, the sp^2 network enables π-π stacking interactions with aromatic structures existent in therapeutic agents, or biomolecules [26]. Finally, pristine graphene has a water contact angle of 95–100° [46] indicative of a hydrophobic nature, which means that therapeutic agents may also establish hydrophobic interactions with graphene via van der Waals interactions. The problem with the extreme hydrophobicity of graphene is the difficulty of dispersing it in aqueous media requiring the use of surfactants or other stabilizing agents to avoid agglomeration in biological fluids [10].

GO preserves unmodified areas of graphene, which are hydrophobic and capable of establishing π–π interactions adequate for drug loading and non-covalent functionalization. However, it can be said that GO has a higher loading potential as it has additional epoxide and hydroxyl groups (**Table 1**) capable of forming hydrogen bonds and weak interactions with other groups of the therapeutic agents [47]. In addition, GO has an amphiphilic nature, since it possesses other oxygen functionalized groups that are ionized at certain pH values (e.g. carboxyl groups are negatively charged at pH values greater than $\approx$4.5) [48]. The presence of ionizable groups and negative charges enhances the reactivity of GO, as additional electrostatic interactions can be established with therapeutic agents. Moreover, charged groups also reduce the water contact angle of GO to 30.7°, improving aqueous solubility and consequently improving colloidal stability [10, 40, 48]. In contrast, rGO (**Table 1**) contains higher number of defects that occurred during GO oxygen removal making it less hydrophobic than graphene (but more hydrophobic than GO) and less reactive than GO [41].

In conclusion, the physicochemical attributes of graphene and rGO make these materials suitable for the loading and delivery of hydrophobic or aromatic bearing therapeutic agents, but their hydrophobic nature creates problems of colloidal stability. In the context of the loading and delivery of therapeutic agents, GO is the GBN that reunites the best physicochemical features: large surface area; capacity of establishing π–π interactions, hydrogen bonds, hydrophobic interactions and electrostatic interactions; amphiphilic nature and colloidal stability [8, 10, 40].

3.4 Optical properties

In terms of electronic transitions, pristine graphene is considered to have a zero-band gap, i.e., no distance between the valence band and the conduction band

[49–51]. This property makes graphene an outstanding electron conductive material, but a material that is unable to reach electronic excited states capable of optical excitation and visible emission. Pristine graphene is also a low-absorption non-photoluminescent material with a 97.7% light transmittance of the total incident light across a wide range of wavelengths [30]. Defect-free or unmodified graphene is therefore not completely suitable for biomedical imaging as its light absorption and optical image contrast are poor. In addition, only when the size of the graphene is reduced to a nanoscale (e.g., in the case of GBNs) can photoluminescence be caused by an increase in the bandgap. In this regard, GO and GQDs are more interesting for biomedical imaging applications due to their intrinsic photoluminescence [49–51]. The bandgap changes that occur during GO reduction decreases rGO photoluminescence capacities.

The origin of GBNs photoluminescence is still widely discussed and not completely elucidated, but three mechanisms have been proposed to explain this property [49–51]:

3.4.1 Quantum confinement effect

In the GBNs structure, the photoluminescent properties are determined by the confinement effect of the π and π^* electronic levels sites of the sp^2 clusters determined by the bandgap of σ and σ^* states of the sp^3 matrix. Upon excitation, an electron from the valence band is promoted to the conduction band leaving a hole behind after absorbing a photon with higher energy than the band-gap energy [50]. This causes the formation of an exciton (a state of excited electron, also referred to as electron–hole pair). When the exciton returns to a lower level this results in the emission of fluorescence [50].

The natural separation distance between the positive charge (hole) and negative charge (electron) in the exciton is designated as the Bohr radius. If the size of the nanomaterial is smaller than the Bohr radius, there will be an electron confinement effect. Excitons have an infinite Bohr radius in graphene. Thus, GBNs, being graphene fragments of any size, will have a quantum confinement effect and, consequently, a photoluminescent effect [50]. GBNs also have a size-dependent photoluminescence as the space between the energy levels (bandgap) can be tuned to the lateral size of the nanomaterial. Smaller sizes have larger band gaps and emit at lower wavelengths, while larger ones have smaller band gaps and emit at higher wavelengths [50].

3.4.2 Surface state

Changing the surface state by the presence of impurities, defects or surface functionalization causes the formation of trap states, i.e., the exciton can be trapped under these conditions leading to a lower-energy radiative emission resulting in a red-shift emission [49–51]. This is what happens, for example, in oxidative graphite exfoliation processes to obtain GO, a process that induces the functionalization of the surface with oxygen functional groups, reducing the band gap energy and therefore causing fluorescence emission at higher wavelengths. This strategy can be used to enhance fluorescent emission in the near infrared (NIR) region known as 'biological window' where the autofluorescence from haemoglobin and biological tissue is negligible and therefore the signal-to-noise ratio can be improved [49–51].

Another proposed mechanism to change emission properties and produce a more emissive material is the creation of conjugated π domain upon a careful choice of the surface functionalization [49–51].

3.4.3 Edges

Depending on the chemical structure of the GBNs edges different emission can be obtained: carbene-like edges have a zig-zag conformation that reduces the band gap energy resulting in a red-shift emission, whereas carbyne like armchair conformation increases the band gap energy resulting in a blue-shift emission [49–51].

Other important optical property that has been exploited for biosensing is the GBNs ability to act as efficient fluorescent quenchers for a variety of fluorophores through nonradiative electronic fluorophore-to-GBN energy transfer.

Finally, a fundamental optical property is the capacity of graphene and its GBNs derivatives to have strong absorption in the NIR range, which means that these nanomaterials are capable of converting photons into heat by NIR irradiation, making them powerful agents for photothermal therapy [52]. In this matter, the reduction of GO to rGO in order to partially restore the aromatic, conjugate character of the graphene sheets increases the absorption of NIR by >6-fold [36].

4. Synthesis of GBNs

Despite the enormous increase in the number of literature studies on graphene synthesis, the large-scale commercial development of graphene is still difficult to achieve [35]. Indeed, the development of cost-effective, highly reliable and scalable synthesis processes with high product yields and quality is a major challenge [35, 53]. In this chapter we will briefly present the methods to synthesize GBNs categorizing these methods in classical and green methods.

4.1 Classical methods

The classical methods (**Figure 1**) used in the synthesis of GBNs can be classified into two categories: top-down and bottom-up [35, 54].

4.1.1 Top-down methods

Top-down methods of GBNs' synthesis start with graphite or other carbon sources such as carbon nanotubes, fullerenes or larger graphene sheets that are cut into smaller monoatomic carbon pieces. These methods may be mechanical, chemical, or physical [55].

One of the most famous mechanical methods is the exfoliation of graphene from graphite firstly described by Geim and Novoselov [1]. This method is remarkably simple and consists of repeatedly gluing a graphite flake with adhesive tape and sticking it and peeling a dozen times [1, 56]. This process can cut a 1 μm thick graphite flake into a single-layer, thin graphene sample that is afterwards transferred to a clean substrate (Si/SiO_2) by gently pressing the tape. Post-heat treatment may be used to remove residues of glue from the tape [37].

Chemical methods range from oxidation processes to other nano-cutting strategies using electrochemical or hydrothermal/solvothermal special oxidation. Oxidation may be handled by a one-or two-step method. The first step uses oxidizing agents (e.g., nitric acid, sulphuric acid, potassium chlorate, potassium permanganate) to oxidize graphite-based materials using the Hummer method or a modified version of the Hummer method [35, 54]. Graphite oxidation breaks the sp^2 hybridized carbon sheets into a graphite sp^2 domain surrounded by sp^3 domains and several defects. Oxidized graphite is a stacked structure similar to graphite, but with a wider spacing between graphite sheets and several oxygen functional groups

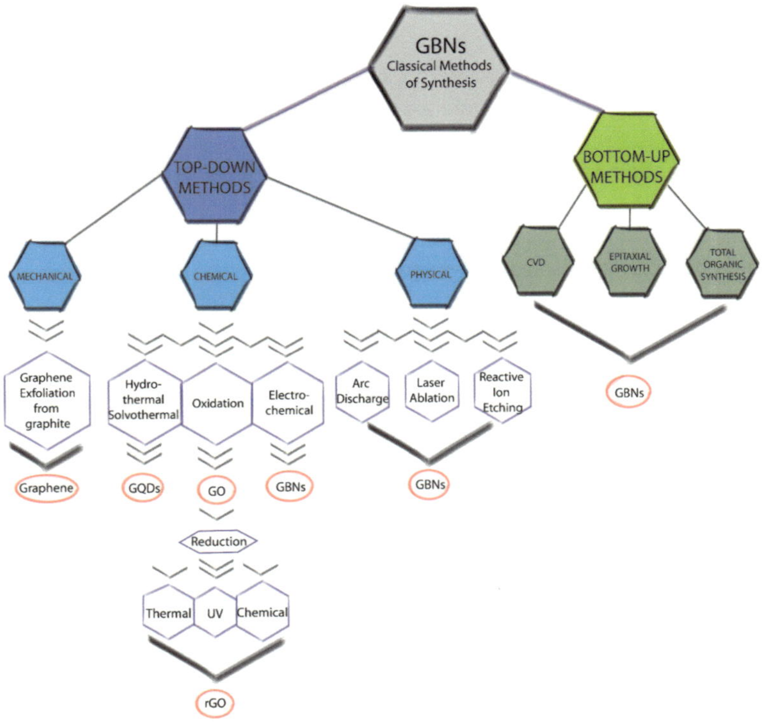

Figure 1.
Classical methods for the synthesis of Graphene-based Nanomaterials (GBNs). Abbreviations: CVD – Carbon Vapor Deposition; GO – Graphene Oxide; rGO – reduced Graphene Oxide; UV – Ultraviolet light.

[35, 54]. In the second step, the oxidized graphite is exfoliated in GO sheets or in smaller parts such as GQDs using mechanical forces in aqueous solutions (sonication and centrifugation) [35, 54]. After obtaining GO sheets, it is possible to remove some of its oxygen functional groups by converting GO to rGO. This can be accomplished by thermal and UV treatment of GO or by chemical reduction using hydrazine, ascorbic acid, sodium borohydride, or hydroquinone [35, 54]. Electrochemical techniques include using chemical agents to assist in the growth of carbon electrodes. Carbon electrodes are broken up by electrochemical cutting, allowing for GBNs to be produced. The applied electric field draws the carbon particles from electrodes through graphite layer intercalation and radical reaction [55]. On the hydrothermal/solvothermal oxidations defect-based carbon materials as GO and carbon nanotubes are cut under high temperature and pressure due to the action of strong alkaline medium. Some special photo-Fenton reactions may also break up GO to form GQDs. Among the physical methods of synthesis, arc discharge, laser ablation or reactive ion etching (RIE) nanolithography are the most widely used. RIE is one of the most efficient for controlling the size and chemical surface of GQDs and is also favorable for the study of some photoluminescent mechanisms [55].

4.1.2 Bottom-up methods

Bottom-up methods are based on the use of simple carbon molecules to build more complex structures such as graphene. These methods include the epitaxial growth of graphene layers on metal carbides by sublimation or by chemical vapor deposition (CVD) directly on metal surfaces [37]. It also includes organic synthesis-based methods in which intramolecular oxidative reactions using polycyclic aromatic hydrocarbons (PAHs) are widely used. Among the bottom-up methods, CVD is the most widely used as it enables low-cost, large-scale production of high-quality materials [37, 55]. The main disadvantages of this method are the high toxicity of the chemical reaction by-product and the need for a fine choice of precursors. CVD production of graphene sheets occurs mainly in two stages [37, 55]. In the first step, the precursor (carbon containing gas) is injected into the reaction chamber. The chamber is subjected to high temperatures and the gas is pyrolyzed inside the chamber to obtain dissociated carbon atoms. This stage must occur on the surface of the substrate to avoid precipitation of carbon clusters during the gaseous phase [37, 55]. The second stage occurs due to the precursor's pyrolysis and corresponds to the deposition of a single atomic layer on the substrate. After the deposition and diffusion of the desired material on the substrate, the by-products dissociate from the substrate and are pumped out of the chamber [37, 55].

Bottom-up methods of synthesis are considered time-consuming and face challenges, therefore focusing on top-down methods that generate GO and rGO are more popular, particularly for the use of GBNs in theranostic applications [54].

4.2 Green methods

As a new category of carbon materials, GBNs have attracted considerable attention due to their tunable photoluminescent properties, low toxicity, strong biocompatibility and excellent photostability [8]. However, despite their general use, standard GBNs' synthetic methods are generally expensive [57], complex and require toxic reagents [58]. The biocompatibility of the carbon content of GBNs may therefore be compromised by the toxicity associated with their classic production methods. Alternatively to classical approaches, GBNs' green approach synthesis, for example, by substituting chemical reducing agents for natural products, is a promising and fascinating field where the resulting material and synthetic processes are biocompatible and can be more safely integrated into living systems for bio-applications [59]. It is therefore important to invest in more sustainable, environmentally friendly, and biocompatible techniques.

Nowadays, various green methods have been reported with interesting applications to produce GBNs alone or conjugated with other substances that enhance their bioactive effect. For example, most of the chemical methods used to date to produce graphene include harsh oxidizers and organic solvents, all of which are environmentally hazardous [60]. Alternatively to chemical methods, green graphene synthesis can be performed by electrochemical exfoliation of graphite into graphene sheets using a molten salt mixture. The molten salts are environmentally friendly and allow the interaction of alkali ions with graphite, which enables the formation of graphene nanosheets and flakes. In addition, this process reduces the number of defects in the graphene structure compared to classic chemical-rich processes [60].

GO's synthesis using classical methods is also very harmful to the environment. For example, in the Hummers method, approximately 1000 times more water than graphite must be used to remove excess oxidants after oxidation reactions, resulting in a large amount of wastewater containing mixed acids and heavy metal ions typically detected on GO sheets [61]. In addition, these methods are all time-consuming, and take a few to hundreds of hours of oxidation. The oxidation time can be shortened to around 1 h simply by using stronger oxidizing mixtures that contribute to further contamination [61]. An alternative green approach to these classical methods is the electrolytic oxidation of graphite water. The GO obtained shows similar chemical composition, structure, and properties to those accomplished by the classical Hummers method and enables ultra-fast oxidation of the graphene lattice within a few seconds, which is more than 100 times faster than currently available methods [61].

The classical synthesis of rGO poses the same problems. The most used reducing agents, such as hydrazine, dimethylhydrazine and sodium borohydride, are highly toxic and remaining trace amounts of these toxic agents can have harmful effects, especially for bio-related applications [62]. In addition, the handling of hazardous waste produced by GO's reduction reaction to the production of rGO may dramatically increase costs on an industrial scale. Efforts have been made over the past few years to counteract toxicity issues by using natural reducing agents [62]. For example, plant extracts (aqueous leaf extracts of *Colocasia esculenta*, *Mesua ferralinn*, *Citrus sinensis*, tea polyphenol [62–65]), microorganisms (bacteria and baker's yeast [62, 66]), amino acids [67], bio-antioxidants (melatonin) [68], non-harmful acids (hydriodic acids, trifluoracetic acid), glucose and glucosamine [62, 69] are used as green reducing agents. Although the degree of reduction of GO by these strategies is typically lower than that of the hydrazine–based method, the excellent biocompatibility of the obtained rGO sheets may enhance their ability to be used in biological and biomedical fields [62].

Preparative methods of GQDs, which are typically manufactured with strong acids or organic solvents, often face severe challenges, and post-treatment with complicated methods remain necessary. Thus, raw materials made from natural renewable resources should be identified, as well as separation and post-treatment procedures that can be performed without complicated processes and without heavy/polluting waste generation [70]. For example, GQDs were synthesized using cotton cellulose, where cellulose and water were part of the reaction mechanism, in the absence of all other dangerous and chemical materials [71]. In another study, GQDs were synthesized by an organic solvent-free methodology using only deionized water and glucose as a precursor [72]. Microwave-assisted synthesis is another technique that has been reported to be able to produce, for example, carbon quantum dots in one-step using roasted chickpeas as carbon source [73] and also aqueous soluble GQDs using cow milk [73]. In another study, GQDs were produced by a simple, eco-friendly and single-pot hydrothermal reaction, with starch as a precursor [74]. In addition, a simple and high-yielding hydrothermal method has been reported to produce GQDs from glucose [75]. GQDs have also been produced using coal tar pitch, a by-product of the coking industries, oxidized with hydrogen peroxide under mild conditions [76]. Finally, also using hydrogen peroxide under mild conditions it is possible to produce GQDs by a greener hydrothermal synthesis using GO as precursor and without involving any harsh reagents [77].

In conclusion, green synthesis of GBNs is an essential area of research that should be promoted within the scientific community once it presents many advantages: (a) it is inexpensive and renewable precursors are easily obtained; (b) it is environmentally-friendly, once no hazardous reagents are needed; (c) it involves simple methods, usually in one-step or one-pot; (d) normally avoids any complicated post-processes [71]; (e) originates products with great biocompatibility [72].

5. Applications of GBNs in therapy and diagnostics (theranostics)

As described earlier, the interesting properties of GBNs have placed these nanomaterials as ideal for creation of theranostic strategies particularly used in the therapy and therapy monitorization (diagnostic) of cancer [8]. Current treatments involve several variations of different strategies that can be used for therapeutic and diagnostic ends. Because each strategy has various inherent advantages and different mechanisms of actuation, a mixture of complementary strategies may result in a synergistic effect. **Figure 2** presents a schematization of the main therapeutic and

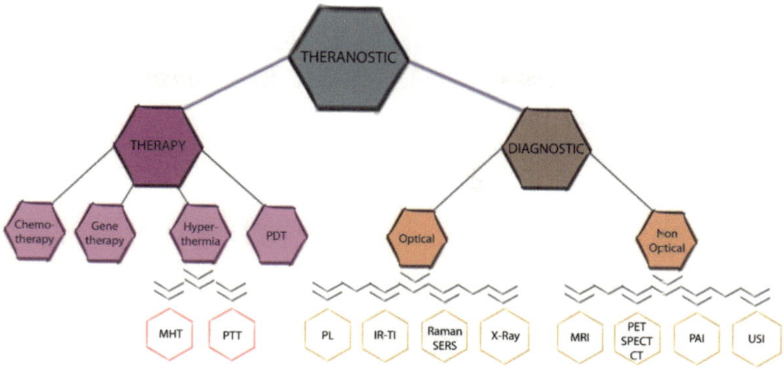

Figure 2.
Theranostic strategies of Graphene-based Nanomaterials. Abbreviations: CT—Computed Tomography; IR-TI—Infrared Thermal Imaging; MHT—Magnetic Hyperthermia Therapy; MRI—Magnetic Resonance Imaging; PAI—Photoacoustic Imaging; PAT—Photoacoustic Therapy; PDT—Photodynamic Therapy; PET—Positron Emission Tomography; PL—Photoluminescence; PTT—Photothermal Therapy; SERS—Super Enhanced Raman Spectroscopy; SPECT—Single Photon Emission Computed Tomography; USI—Ultrasound Imaging.

diagnostic strategies. The therapeutic and diagnostic strategies of GBNs will be presented together with some examples of their use in the following subsections.

5.1 Therapeutic strategies

5.1.1 Chemotherapy and gene therapy

The GBNs' intrinsic properties have paved the way for the advancement of approaches to chemotherapy and gene therapy.

Chemotherapy implies the use of anticancer drugs which, by several mechanisms (i.e., interfering with angiogenesis and cell division), may result in cellular damage/stress and may lead to cell death if apoptosis is triggered. The chemotherapeutic arsenal is widely known as it is the basis of classical cancer therapy [8]. Furthermore, by incorporating these drugs into nanocarriers like GBNs, the toxic effects of anticancer drugs in healthy cells that are not affected by cancer can be reduced [8]. Indeed, GBNs (especially GO) have a high drug loading ratio of hydrophilic and lipophilic anticancer drugs, due to the combination of a large surface area and the presence of delocalized π electrons, as well as chemical polar groups [8]. The diverse range of potential chemical interactions between anticancer drugs and GBNs has conferred to these nanocarriers an important role in chemotherapy, as drug loading ratios can exceed 200 wt%, which is unusually high compared to other nanocarriers [78]. For example, the commercial liposomal formulations Caelyx® and Doxil® containing the anticancer drug doxorubicin have a drug load of 16 wt %, while the majority of GBNs' formulations can meet the drug loading values from 55 wt % to 133 wt % [79–85]. GBNs loaded with another anticancer drug, paclitaxel, also achieved a remarkably effective drug loading of 90 wt % compared to commercial formulations containing this drug: Taxol® and Abraxane® with a drug loading of 1 wt % and 11 wt %, respectively [86].

Gene therapy requires the incorporation of genes, gene segments or oligonucleotides in nanocarriers that provide protection against enzyme-induced degradation and/or inactivation of the genetic material [8, 87]. When used in cancer, the mechanism of action of this therapeutic strategy is based on: (i) deactivation of oncogenes; (ii) substitution of non-functioning tumor suppressor genes; (iii) inducing cell death or repair of normal cell function; (iv) defense of normal cells from drug-induced toxicity or activation of immune cells for the destruction of cancer cells [8, 87]. The same favorable properties of GBNs for chemotherapy are valid for explaining their use in gene therapy. Indeed, GBNs have shown the ability to efficiently condense genetic material by π-π stacking interactions, avoiding endonuclease's degradation of nucleic acids [40, 88, 89].

5.1.2 Hyperthermia

Hyperthermia is a therapeutic strategy that causes the temperature rise to kill cancer cells. Mild hyperthermia (temperature rise to 43–50°C) induces increased membrane permeability, defective membrane transport, metabolic signaling disturbance leading to cell apoptosis. Extreme hyperthermia (temperature rise >50°C) causes necrotic cell death due to cell membrane disruption and protein denaturation [8].

The optical and thermal properties of GBNs make these nanosystems desirable for their use in the hyperthermia treatment of cancer cells. GBNs have a wide absorption in the NIR region (700–1100 nm) and can convert it into thermal energy causing local hyperthermia. At the same time, the hyperthermia effect can reduce GBNs' oxygen functional groups causing the release of gas. The formation and collapse of gas bubbles contributes to the development of a microcavitation environment often responsible for the death of cancer cells. Hyperthermia therapy strategy, based on the conversion of absorbed NIR to thermal energy, is known as photothermal therapy (PTT) [8, 90, 91]. Over the last 6 years, PTT has been the therapeutic strategy most explored by researchers working with GBNs [83, 92–97]. This is primarily because this strategy has the advantage of not needing cell internalization of GBNs while maintaining a deep penetration of biological tissues [8]. The efficacy of PTT to destroy cancer cells has also been improved by conjugation of GBNs with other narrow-bandgap materials [84, 85, 98–112]. Moreover, while GO has been the perfect GBN for chemotherapy and gene therapy, rGO is the preferred nanomaterial for PTT because it has an NIR absorption 6 times higher than GO [8, 113].

Another strategy to increase the death of cancer cells by hyperthermia is to combine magnetic hyperthermia (MHT) with PTT through conjugation of GBNs with magnetic nanoparticles (MNPs) [82, 113]. MNPs exposed to an external alternating magnetic field can convert magnetic energy into thermal energy by Néel or Brownian relaxation mechanisms. When the application of the magnetic field is faster than the relaxation time of the MNPs, the delay in magnetic moment relaxation induces MHT [8].

5.1.3 Photodynamic therapy

Recently, GBNs have also been applied to photodynamic therapy (PDT) strategy used to kill cancer cells [8, 52, 114]. This strategy requires a photosensitizer (PS) agent to be loaded into the GBNs by π-π stacking and/or hydrophobic interactions. Upon photon absorption, the PS agent will be excited to a singlet state after which it decays into a low-energy excited triplet state through intersystem crossing. Then, in the excited triplet state, PS transfers an electron to: (i) different molecules producing reactive oxygen species (ROS): $O_2^{\bullet -}$, H_2O_2, $HO^{\bullet}$or (ii) oxygen originating $^1O_2$. ROS interact with cellular components of cancer cells (lipids, proteins, nucleic acids) causing oxidative stress and ultimately cell death [8, 52, 114].

PDT is commonly used in conjunction with PTT to benefit from the synergistic influence of both therapeutic strategies [101, 108, 115–124].

5.2 Diagnostic strategies

5.2.1 Photoluminescence

GBNs possess attractive optical features applied to the monitoring of therapeutic efficacy. As a result, GBNs act as dye-free labeling to follow the delivery of therapeutic nanosystems to cells. Due to the quantum confinement effect that exists when the sizes of GBNs are smaller than their exciton Bohr radii, the nano-sized material has non-blinking photoluminescence (PL) and photostability [8]. GBNs therefore emit low-energy fluorescence when excited by high-energy light (usually UV or visible light) and GBNs' fluorescence intensity remains strong under confocal laser lighting. GQDs are among the most used GBNs for their PL [88, 89, 99, 115, 125–129].

Upon conjugation of GBNs with upconversion luminescence nanoparticles (UCNPs), such as: $NaYF_4$:Yb^{3+}, Er^{3+} or $NaYF_4$: Yb^{3+}, Tm^{3+} an anti-Stoke emission occurs when two or more low-energy photons from NIR light are absorbed to generate higher energy emissions in the visible region. The conjugation with UCNPs confers to GBNs an even more fascinating PL property, as in this case excitation with NIR light produces emission at lower wavelengths. The advantages of this upconversion PL are due to the use of NIR light excitation, which reduces autofluorescence of biological tissues and increases penetration depths, thus reducing photo-damage of healthy tissues [8, 95, 101, 121, 124].

The fluorescence quenching capability demonstrated by GBNs resulting from fluorescence resonance energy transfer (FRET) or non-radiative dipole–dipole interactions between fluorescence species and GBNs is also important. The fluorescence quenching effect is used as an external diagnostic feature that enables the release of GBNs' cargo to be identified [8]. Indeed, when GBNs interact with fluorescent cargo (drugs or other active substances) they reduce their fluorescence emission, but when the cargo is released, the fluorescence emission is reset [79, 130].

5.2.2 Infrared thermal imaging

Infrared thermal imaging (IR-TI) is a diagnostic strategy based on thermal changes due to radiation absorption. Light absorbed and not lost by emission results in heat that can be registered as an image [8]. As a result, the GBNs photothermal conversion properties used in PTT can also be used as a therapy-guiding strategy under an IR-TI non-labelling technique. The use of the NIR laser to trigger a PTT effect can be detected by means of a visible thermal field signal, which is especially important because of its non-invasive nature and because it provides real-time images [8]. Provided that PTT is one of the treatment modalities most commonly used by GBN-producing researchers for biomedical applications, IR-TI is also widely used, as both strategies (PTT and IR-TI) are often used together [92–99, 105–108, 110, 112, 113, 119, 120, 124, 131–133].

5.2.3 Raman spectroscopy and surface enhanced Raman spectroscopy

Raman scattering-based spectroscopy can be used as a diagnostic technique to obtain morphological and chemical information from accessible tissue surfaces, e.g., skin, gastrointestinal tract, or intraoperatively. This imaging technique combines the surface imaging of the tissues with the Raman spectra provided by its molecular components [8]. When visible or NIR light interacts with the surface material it originates inelastic scattering of photons (Raman scattering) that display a shift in frequency. The energy shift provides information on the vibrational modes in the system. GBNs usually demonstrate the required Raman scattering intensity, exhibiting the standard D, G and 2-D band characteristics of the vibrational modes in the range 1000–3000 cm^{-1}. As a result, the delivery of GBNs used as cancer therapeutic tools can be followed by Raman imaging of the tissues [8].

Raman imaging is an even more effective diagnostic strategy when GBNs are associated with gold and silver nanoparticles. In this case, the Raman signals of GBNs are significantly improved by the surface enhanced Raman scattering (SERS). Indeed, SERS occurs when molecules are adsorbed or located near a metallic nanostructure, i.e., the improvement of the Raman scattering occurs due to the resonant interaction of light with the surface plasmons that are excited at the surface of the metallic nanostructure. Using this strategy, SERS can be used to combine microscope cell imaging with Raman spectroscopy, mapping the presence of GBNs in the tumor tissue of the cell [8, 103].

5.2.4 Ultrasound Imaging

Using the electrical properties of GBNs, it is possible to image these nanosystems in their journey through the body using ultrasound imaging (USI) strategies [96, 102]. USI is therefore based on the conversion of electrical signals to ultrasound waves that penetrate the body and biological tissues. Some of these ultrasound waves are reflected and transformed by a transducer into electrical signals that are handled and displayed as an image [8].

5.2.5 Photoacoustic imaging

Photoacoustic Imaging (PAI) is another diagnostic strategy that benefits from the NIR absorption capacity of GBNs and enables monitoring their distribution in body tissues. When tissues are irradiated with NIR short laser pulses, locally dispersed GBNs absorb energy and generate heat that leads to thermoelastic expansion followed by contraction and consequent emission of mechanical pressure waves at ultrasonic frequencies [8]. Periodic sound waves produced can be sensed by ultrasonic transducers creating an image by mapping the original absorbed energy distribution [8]. Among the GBNs, rGO has gained interest as a PAI contrast agent due to its higher NIR absorbance properties [85, 96, 125, 134]. In spite of the improved PAI properties of rGO, GO nanomaterials compensate for their lower NIR absorption with higher loading capacity. In some studies, thus, GO nanomaterials were loaded with other narrow-band gap materials as a solution to increase NIR absorption and thus also attained PAI diagnostic modality [80, 100, 105, 110].

5.2.6 Tomography

Tomography is a nuclear medicine imaging technique where a cyclotron is used to produce short or ultra-short-lived radionuclides that decay with the emission of: (i) positron, in the case of Positron Emission Tomography (PET); (ii) γ rays in the case of Single Photon Emission Computed Tomography (SPECT); and multiple X-rays in the case of Computed Tomography (CT). All these techniques rely on differential levels of the radiation attenuation within the body to create three-dimensional, high-contrast anatomical images that allow for delineation between various structures [8].

The physicochemical properties of GBNs promote the loading of these nanocarriers with radionuclides that enable tomography imaging of tissues [85, 102, 124, 132].

5.2.7 Magnetic resonance imaging

Magnetic resonance imaging (MRI) consists of the application of radiofrequency pulses and is derived from the interaction between the water protons and the magnetic field applied. The resulting image is produced by the pattern of absorption and emission of the electromagnetic wave [8]. In order to increase the visibility of anatomical structures, contrast agents (MRI probes) are used to reduce the relaxation times of water protons inside body tissues [8]. The unusual wide surface area and high loading capacity of the GBNs have also proven to be very advantageous for carrying MRI probes [81–83, 113, 124, 130]. In addition, the high molecular weight of GBNs can reduce the rotational motion of the water proton, increase the relaxation time and increase the *in vivo* half-life of the MRI contrast agent, resulting in a better image [113].

6. Application of GBNs in bioremediation

GBNs offer a holistic approach to health. In fact, in the previous sections, we described the great potential of GBNs in human health due to their role in therapy and diagnosis. Moreover, GBNs or their functionalized derivatives are cutting-edge materials used in bioremediation, and their remarkable properties can be used to mitigate environmental contaminants, as well as to improve human, plant, and animal health [17–20, 25, 135].

The following sections describe the properties of GBNs that favor their use in bioremediation and the major pollutants on which GBNs have demonstrated their bioremediation efficiency.

6.1 GBNs properties and processes involved in bioremediation

Graphene oxidation to GO and rGO reinforces its properties and improves its hydrophilic nature, thereby enhancing its ability to associate with contaminants either physically or chemically. This association can be processed by adsorption of contaminants on the surface of GBNs or by the oxidation breakdown of contaminants, by photocatalysis or other advanced oxidation processes (AOPs) [18].

6.1.1 Adsorption

One of the most widely used processes for bioremediation is chemical and physical adsorption. The adsorption capacity of materials depends on several characteristics [25]:

i. good mechanical strength for handling and possibly regenerating and reusing;

ii. strong wettability to ensure use in the adsorption of water pollutants;

iii. high porosity in favor of physical adsorption;

iv. large surface area and different functional groups to promote chemical adsorption.

As previously described GBNs obey to all these requirements and hold great potential as adsorbent materials. GBNs have a large surface area and excellent mechanical properties. GBNs also have favorable wettability and different functional surface and edge groups (in these aspects GO has more adsorbent properties than rGO) [18]. As far as porosity is concerned, highly porous GBNs have recently been developed by chemical activation of GO precursors with KOH [25]. Other GBN derivatives functionalized with metal/oxide composites or magnetic nanoparticles may also improve the adsorption capacity of GBNs or demonstrate advantages in the magnetic separation of contaminants adsorbed and re-use of adsorbents by adsorption–desorption cycles [20, 25, 135]. GBNs can also be functionalized with chelating compounds like ethylenediamine tetraacetic acid (EDTA) which favors adsorption of metal ions [19]. However, while the functionalization of GBNs may improve the adsorption capacity of some specific contaminant, it may also limit its use for a more generic type of adsorbate [20].

With regard to the chemical versatility of GBNs, this material is certainly advantageous in comparison with other adsorbents [15, 19, 20]. For example, GO has oxygen-functionalized groups (e.g., COOH) which are deprotonated at a broad range of pH values ($\approx$ pH > 4.5) and therefore negatively charged groups establish electrostatic interactions with cationic pollutants [19]. Oxygen-functionalized groups also enable hydrogen bonding with adsorbate compounds. These interactions may be established between hydrogen with a partial positive charge and an electronegative atom such as chlorine, fluorine, or oxygen [20]. Hydrogen bonding can therefore be formed between hydrogen atoms present in the functional moieties of GBNs and partially negatively charged atoms of the adsorbate molecule [20]. Hydrophobic interaction is driven by the entropic effect that occurs when ordered water molecules are banned from nonpolar carbon surface of GBNs. Hydrophobic interaction is also another significant contribution to the adsorption of hydrophobic/amphiphilic contaminants to GBNs [19]. Finally, GBNs have the possibility to establish π-π interactions with aromatic rings from contaminants, which may be the only interaction established or may be strengthened by simultaneous electrostatic interactions in cases where aromatic contaminants are also charged [19, 20].

Figure 3 illustrates the possible adsorption mechanisms of the different pollutant compounds on GBN adsorbents.

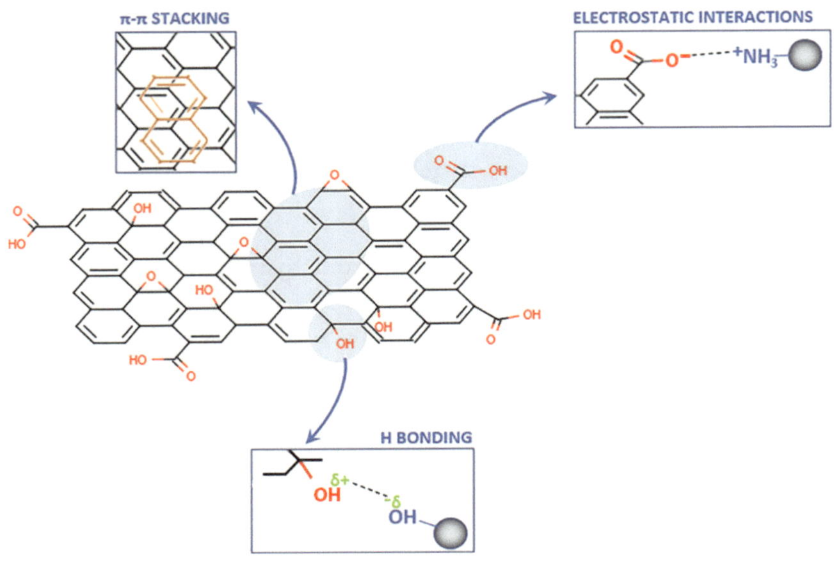

Figure 3.
Common chemical interactions established between Graphene-based Nanomaterials and pollutants.

6.1.2 Oxidation and photocatalysis

GO-presenting oxygen functional groups also lead to redox reactions and make different contaminants environmentally friendly and degradable [18]. This removes the problem of waste management that exists in the case of adsorption. Radical-based oxidation processes, also referred to as AOPs, specifically turn organic entities into environmentally compatible harmless entities, including various minerals, less toxic fragments of carbon-based contaminants, and neutral entities such as water and carbon dioxide [18]. Photocatalysis is also an AOP that is effective in the degradation of various organic pollutants by GBNs and their composites. GBNs with a zero-band gap are capable of absorbing light over a wide spectrum. This allows the electrons to be excited from the valence band to the conduction band, forming holes in the valence band. Both electrons and holes are involved in redox reactions that produce many radicals (e.g., hydroxyl radicals) [18]. These radicals serve as potent oxidizers across the surface of GBNs and are responsible for photocatalysis of organic contaminants enabling the destruction of dyes and other organic matter from wastewater [18]. It is also helpful to reduce the band gap of GBNs by loading them with materials such as titanium (TiO_2) and zinc oxide (ZnO) to allow efficient use of solar irradiation during photocatalytic decomposition [17].

6.2 Atmospheric pollutants

6.2.1 Gas pollutants

Gas pollutants have risen over decades due to industrial developments and have become one of the most significant issues in the modern world. Because of its widespread combustion from vehicles, forest fires and manufacturing processes, CO_2 is the air pollutant of most concern [20]. The ability to block infrared irradiation in the stratospheric layer exacerbates the greenhouse effect and, thus, global warming [20]. Chlorofluorocarbon (CFC), a gas used in freezers, refrigerators, and air-conditioners, is another chemical specie which causes serious damage to the atmosphere. CFC has the property of interacting with ozone causing damage to the ozone layer, responsible for filtering UV irradiation from sunlight [20]. Inorganic gaseous pollutants such as SO_2, NO_2, NH_3 and H_2S are also implicated in the phenomenon of acid rain [20, 25]. Monuments and buildings damage, flora degradation, a reduction in soil pH, pollution of the bodies of water and human diseases are the environmental effects of acid rain in large cities; however, it is very difficult to measure them economically [20]. In addition, possible health hazards such as respiratory irritation and damage to the central nervous system have been associated with long-term exposure to these contaminants [20].

GO and other GBNs as well as their modified forms are good adsorbents for the reactive removal of these toxic gases. Most of the research, however, concentrated on NH_3 adsorption using GBNs and composites modified by metal oxide. Owing to the presence of diverse active defect sites, such as the hydroxyl and epoxy functional groups and their neighboring carbon atoms, NH_3 adsorption on GO is usually greater than that on other GBNs [25].

6.2.2 Volatile organic compounds

A wide number of volatile organic compounds (VOCs) are responsible for the growth of cancer in people all over the world, according to the WHO [20]. Formaldehyde which comes from paint and decorating materials, is one of VOCs and the major indoor air pollutant responsible for the sick building syndrome [25].

In order to reduce harm to the environment and human health caused by VOCs, GBNs, in particular GO, have recently been employed in several studies for VOC removal by adsorption and photocatalytic decomposition [20, 25].

6.3 Water pollutants

One of the long-lasting concerns in the past few decades has been aquatic contamination due to industrial activities. Groundwater, surface water and wastewater systems contain many pollutants [14, 17, 20, 25]. Anions and heavy metal cations as well as organic compounds are significant contaminants (e.g., dye from textile factories, pesticides, and pharmaceuticals) [14, 17, 20, 21, 25]. Aqueous pollutants arising from waste oil from numerous oil leakage incidents and eventually from biological contaminants may also be identified [17, 20].

6.3.1 Inorganic metals and metalloid cations

Owing to their high toxicity to plants, animals and human beings, heavy metals are the most substantial contaminants in water. The most prevalent heavy metals in contaminated waters are Hg, Pb, Ag, Cu, Cd, Cr, Zn, Ni, Co and Mn [21, 25]. Most metal ions are found in cationic forms, but certain metals are present in anions such as Cr (VI) within CrO_4^{2-}, $Cr_2O_7^{2-}$ [21, 25]. The most important metalloid ion with high toxicity is arsenic present in the form of As (V) in $H_2AsO_4^-$ and $HAsO4^{2-}$ [135]. Arsenic is frequently present in soils and rocks in the form of minerals that are mobilized into groundwater by natural weathering, geochemical reactions, biological activity, volcanic emissions and industrial activities [135]. The high degree of exposure to arsenic by water is a calamity for developing countries. More than 100 million people from densely populated countries, including Bangladesh, China, India, Pakistan, Taiwan, and Mexico, and more than 70% of people from Asian continents, live at risk of arsenic-contaminated ground water and are drinking potable water contaminated with excessive levels of arsenic [25]. Huge amounts of adverse problems are caused by exposure to elevated concentrations of arsenic from drinking water and are commonly associated with skin lesions and hyperkeratosis as adverse effects, whereas long-term exposure leads to cancers of the skin, kidneys, liver and prostate. In addition, arsenic also affects nervous and cardiovascular system functions [25, 135].

Adsorption is probably the most efficient way to eliminate aquatic heavy metal ions, because bioprocessing and chemical reactions like photocatalysis are unable to destroy the metal ions. Due to the numerous functional groups on the surface, GO is a potential adsorbent for metal ion complexation by both electrostatic and coordination methods (e.g., upon GO functionalization with EDTA) [25]. Arsenic removal has become imperative, but most treatment processes are expensive, except for adsorption, which is affordable, convenient and easy to handle. For water treatment, GO and its composite-based membranes, thin films, paper-like materials, and solid composite materials have gained notoriety and have shown efficient and high potential for arsenic removal [135, 136]. The numerous oxygen functional groups are responsible for both higher adsorption and desorption potential of GO. With a change in solvent pH, arsenic desorption from the GO surface contributes to GO regeneration, which can be used to repeat adsorption–desorption processes, thus increasing adsorption efficiency and reducing costs [135]. The adsorption capability, selectivity, thermal and chemical stability of GO can be enhanced by surface modifications. Moreover, conjugation of GO with magnetic nanoparticles also facilitates the magneto-responsive separation of depleted adsorbents from water [135].

6.3.2 Inorganic anions

Some inorganic anions, F^-, NO_3^-, SO_4^{2-}, ClO_4^-, PO_4^{3-}, are still found in large amounts in water, and they may also cause water pollution and should be removed, although they are less harmful than heavy metal ions [25]. The presence of large amounts of NO_3^- and PO_4^{3-}, in water, for instance, can induce eutrophication (i.e., water enriched with nutrients that induce excessive growth of algae). Due to the negative anion charge, GO is not so successful for inorganic anion adsorption [25]. GBNs and functionalized GBNs, however, have been identified as efficient in inorganic anion adsorption. For example, the surface exchange between F^- in solution and hydroxyl ions promotes the adsorption of these anions to GBNs [25, 137].

6.3.3 Organic pollutants: dyes, polycyclic aromatic hydrocarbons, pesticides, and pharmaceuticals

Dyes are a class of organic compounds commonly found as water contaminants that are released from a wide variety of sources, such as printing, textiles, dyeing, paper production, tanning, and painting industries. Most dyes are durable and difficult to biodegrade and have complex molecular structures. By altering the color of water, the presence of dyes in water causes disturbance of the photosynthetic phase of aquatic plants, thus suppressing sunshine, creating an imbalance in the entire aquatic environment [18, 25]. In addition, certain dyes are detrimental to human beings. Most dyes are dissolved in water and are either cationic or anionic. By establishing electrostatic interactions, GO exhibits high adsorption of cationic dyes, but between GO anionic groups and anionic dyes, there is strong electrostatic repulsion. However, because of additional π-π stacking interactions, GBNs and composites can still be excellent adsorbents for cationic and anionic dyes [18, 25].

Another class of organic pollutants composed of repeated aromatic ring structures is polycyclic aromatic hydrocarbons (PAHs) [18]. They are non-charged and non-polar molecules produced from different methods, such as petroleum products burning, incomplete biomass combustion, coal mining [18], etc. PAHs have adverse effects on human health and are believed to cause cancer of the skin, blood, bladder, liver and cardiovascular diseases [18]. Owing to insufficient waste management, leakage and accidents, monocyclic aromatic hydrocarbons such as toluene, xylene, benzene are also largely excreted from industry causing damage to the human central nervous system [18].

Many pesticides are organic aromatic compounds still commonly used in agriculture, dairy, and insect control. In addition, pesticides have also been used in domestic gardening and veterinary practice by common citizens. Therefore, the systematic usage of pesticides is of concern owing to their neurotoxicity, carcinogenic potential and involvement in other pathologies [20, 138]. Moreover, the toxicity of organophosphorus pesticides lies in the fact that these compounds are inhibitors of acetylcholinesterase enzymes, which contribute to dysfunction of the nervous system [20].

Pharmaceutical drugs are also organic contaminants that have harmful effects on the environment and human health. Even at low concentrations, these chemicals are very difficult to remove and between 30 and 90% remain undegradable and are excreted as active compounds in the environment [20, 135].

Numerous investigations have demonstrated potential in the use of GO and other GBNs for the adsorption of PAHs, phenolic compounds, pesticides, and pharmaceutical drugs [20, 21, 25, 39, 135, 138]. In general, there are five potential interactions, including hydrophobic effects, π-π stacking, hydrogen bonds, and covalent and electrostatic interactions, which are assumed to be responsible for the adsorption of organic compounds on the GBNs' surface [15, 19, 20, 25] (**Figure 3**). In the case of GO and other GBNs, the majority of investigations have shown that π-π association plays an important role in the adsorption of aromatic organic contaminants [25]. In comparison, the latest major methods used to treat these pollutants are AOPs and the chemical-microbial depletion [20].

6.3.4 Oil and its derivatives

The significant rise in the discovery of crude oil and the increase in the production of petroleum derivatives have caused negative and long-term destruction of various habitats [20]. One of the most important pollution issues happening very frequently in the ocean or seashore is oil leakage from reservoirs, ships, or oil drilling facilities. In order to minimize the harmful impact on marine ecology, the adsorption of leaking oils from polluted seawater has been an important area of study [17]. Latest experiments have successfully investigated the adsorption of oil emulsions on GBNs, demonstrating excellent adsorption capacities. Extremely porous GBNs (sponges, hydrogels and xerogels) are recently developed as cutting-edge oil adsorbents; many of them are conjugated with magnetic metallic nanospheres and typically have high recyclability [17, 20].

6.3.5 Biological contaminants

A significant process for public health safety is also the disinfection of the water supply and indoor air to remove common harmful pathogens, like bacteria (e.g., *E. coli*, *F. Solani*), and viruses (e.g., EV71 and H9N2 virus). In these cases, the use of GBNs together with UVC light is also effective for decontamination by photocatalysis [17].

7. Conclusions and prospects

In this chapter, the current progress on the use of various GBNs in the treatment of cancer and bioremediation has been reviewed. The extraordinary properties of GBNs have also been described with special focus in those that favor the biomedical applications of this material, i.e., the large surface area, the large number of unsaturated π-bonds, the mechanical strength, the NIR absorption properties, the PL capacity, etc. The versatility of GBNs is indicated as a feature that can be explored in the most diverse biomedical fields. In this sense, the use of GBNs in cancer theranostic strategies has been discussed. Successful research studies using GBNs for the loading of anticancer drugs or nucleic acids in synergistic chemotherapy, gene therapy and photothermal/photodynamic therapy have been revised in the field of cancer therapy. GBNs have also been described as imaging diagnostic tools used to track the path of therapeutic delivery in target tissues. Finally, the application of GBNs for photocatalysis and adsorption was described as a means of environmental decontamination, i.e., bioremediation.

It is clear from all the revised research that GBNs have a great future in biomedical applications, either as therapeutic tools or as bioremediation strategies, where specifically GO can be considered one of the most advanced and promising adsorbents. However, despite successful attempts to use GBNs in the biomedical field, there are still several challenges that need to be overcome prior to their widespread commercial or clinical use. First, green methods must be used to develop environmentally sustainable approaches to the production of GBNs. Some attempts at green synthesis have been made, but they are still far from proposing standard and reproducible methods that can be scaled up to reduce production costs while maintaining a minimal presence of residual contaminants. In addition, although many studies have shown that GBN's adsorbents have been recycled, these studies are still scarce and more innovative research work needs to be explored in the future to achieve convenient separation and regeneration of GBN's adsorbents.

Acknowledgements

This work was supported by Fundação para a Ciência e Tecnologia (FCT) in the framework of the Strategic Funding Funding [UID/FIS/04650/2019], and by the project CONCERT [POCI-01-0145-FEDER-032651 and PTDC/NAN-MAT/326512017], co-financed by the European Regional Development Fund (ERDF), through COMPETE 2020, under Portugal 2020, and FCT I.P. M Lúcio thanks FCT and ERDF for doctoral position [CTTI-150/18-CF (1)] in the ambit of the project CONCERT. Eduarda Fernandes acknowledges FCT for PhD grant (SFRH/BD/147938/2019).

Abbreviations

AOPs	Advanced oxidation processes
CFC	Chlorofluorocarbon
CSCs	Cancer stem cells
CVD	Chemical vapor deposition
CT	Computed Tomography
EDTA	Ethylenediamine tetraacetic acid
FRET	Fluorescence resonance energy transfer
GBNs	Graphene-based nanomaterials
GQDs	Graphene quantum dots
GO	Graphene oxide
rGO	Reduced graphene oxide
IARC	International Agency for Research on Cancer
IR-TI	Infrared Thermal Imaging
MHT	Magnetic Hyperthermia Therapy
MNPs	Magnetic nanoparticles
MRI	Magnetic Resonance Imaging
NIR	Near infrared
PAHs	Polycyclic aromatic hydrocarbons
PAI	Photoacoustic Imaging
PAT	Photoacoustic Therapy
PDT	Photodynamic Therapy
PET	Positron Emission Tomography
PL	Photoluminescence
PS	Photosensitizer
PTT	Photothermal Therapy
RIE	Reactive ion etching
ROS	Reactive oxygen species
SERS	Super Enhanced Raman Spectroscopy
SPECT	Single Photon Emission Computed Tomography
UCNPs	Upconversion luminescence nanoparticles
USI	Ultrasound Imaging
VOCs	Volatile organic compounds
WHO	World Health Organization

Author details

Marlene Lúcio[1,2]*, Eduarda Fernandes[1], Hugo Gonçalves[3], Sofia Machado[2], Andreia C. Gomes[2,4] and Maria Elisabete C.D. Real Oliveira[1]

1 Departamento de Física da Universidade do Minho, CF-UM-UP, Centro de Física das Universidades do Minho e Porto, Braga, Portugal

2 Departamento de Biologia, CBMA, Centro de Biologia Molecular e Ambiental, Universidade do Minho, Braga, Portugal

3 Paralab, SA, Valbom, Portugal

4 IB-S, Institute of Science and Innovation for Bio-Sustainability, Portugal

*Address all correspondence to: mlucio@fisica.uminho.pt

References

[1] Novoselov KS, Geim AK, Morozov SV, Jiang D, Zhang Y, Dubonos SV, Grigorieva IV, Firsov AA. Electric Field Effect in Atomically Thin Carbon Films. Science. 2004;306(5696): 666-669. DOI:10.1126/science.1102896

[2] Castro Neto AH, Guinea F, Peres NMR, Novoselov KS, Geim AK. The electronic properties of graphene. Reviews of Modern Physics. 2009;81(1): 109-162. DOI:10.1103/RevModPhys. 81.109

[3] Wang F, Shi S. Optical Properties of Graphene. In: Avouris P, Low T, Heinz TF, editors. 2D Materials: Properties and Devices. Cambridge: Cambridge University Press; 2017. p. 38-51. DOI:10.1017/9781316681619.004

[4] Allen MJ, Tung VC, Kaner RB. Honeycomb Carbon: A Review of Graphene. Chemical Reviews. 2010;110 (1):132-145. DOI:10.1021/cr900070d

[5] Randviir EP, Brownson DAC, Banks CE. A decade of graphene research: production, applications and outlook. Materials Today. 2014;17(9): 426-432. DOI:10.1016/j. mattod.2014.06.001

[6] Aïssa B, Memon NK, Ali A, Khraisheh MK. Recent Progress in the Growth and Applications of Graphene as a Smart Material: A Review. Frontiers in Materials. 2015;2(58). DOI:10.3389/ fmats.2015.00058

[7] Sood AK, Lund I, Puri YR, Efstathiadis H, Haldar P, Dhar NK, Lewis J, Dubey M, Zakar E, Wijewarnasuriya P, Polla DL, Fritze M. Review of Graphene Technology and Its Applications for Electronic Devices. In: Ebrahimi F, editor. Graphene - New Trends and Developments. Available from: https://www.intechopen.com/ books/graphene-new-trends-and-developments/review-of-graphene-technology-and-its-applications-for-electronic-devices: IntechOpen; 2015. DOI:10.5772/61316

[8] Viseu T, Lopes CM, Fernandes E, Oliveira MECDR, Lúcio M. A Systematic Review and Critical Analysis of the Role of Graphene-Based Nanomaterials in Cancer Theranostics. Pharmaceutics. 2018;10(4):282. DOI:10.3390/ pharmaceutics10040282

[9] Reina G, González-Domínguez JM, Criado A, Vázquez E, Bianco A, Prato M. Promises, facts and challenges for graphene in biomedical applications. Chemical Society Reviews. 2017;46(15): 4400-4416. DOI:10.1039/C7CS00363C

[10] Goenka S, Sant V, Sant S. Graphene-based nanomaterials for drug delivery and tissue engineering. Journal of Controlled Release. 2014;173:75-88. DOI: 10.1016/j.jconrel.2013.10.017

[11] Kim MG, Park JY, Shon Y, Shim G, Oh YK. Pharmaceutical applications of graphene-based nanosheets. Curr Pharm Biotechnol. 2014;14(12): 1016-1026. DOI: 10.2174/ 1389201015666140113113222

[12] Yang K, Feng L, Shi X, Liu Z. Nano-graphene in biomedicine: theranostic applications. Chem Soc Rev. 2013;42(2): 530-547. DOI:10.1039/c2cs35342c

[13] Chen Y, Tan C, Zhang H, Wang L. Two-dimensional graphene analogues for biomedical applications. Chem Soc Rev. 2015;44(9):2681-2701. DOI: 10.1039/c4cs00300d

[14] Kommu A, Singh JK. A review on graphene-based materials for removal of toxic pollutants from wastewater. Soft Materials. 2020:1-26. DOI:10.1080/ 1539445x.2020.1739710

[15] Kim S, Park CM, Jang M, Son A, Her N, Yu M, Snyder S, Kim D-H,

Yoon Y. Aqueous removal of inorganic and organic contaminants by graphene-based nanoadsorbents: A review. Chemosphere. 2018;212:1104-1124. DOI: 10.1016/j.chemosphere.2018.09.033

[16] Lü K, Zhao G, Wang X. A brief review of graphene-based material synthesis and its application in environmental pollution management. Chinese Science Bulletin. 2012;57(11): 1223-1234. DOI:10.1007/s11434-012-4986-5

[17] Tsang CHA, Kwok HYH, Cheng Z, Leung DYC. The applications of graphene-based materials in pollutant control and disinfection. Progress in Solid State Chemistry. 2017;45-46:1-8. DOI: 10.1016/j.progsolidstchem.2017.02.001

[18] Thakur K, Kandasubramanian B. Graphene and Graphene Oxide-Based Composites for Removal of Organic Pollutants: A Review. Journal of Chemical & Engineering Data. 2019;64(3):833-867. DOI:10.1021/acs.jced.8b01057

[19] Xu J, Lv H, Yang S-T, Luo J. Preparation of graphene adsorbents and their applications in water purification. Reviews in Inorganic Chemistry. 2013; 33(2-3):139-160. DOI:10.1515/revic-2013-0007

[20] Fraga TJM, Carvalho MN, Ghislandi MG, Motta Sobrinho MA. Functionalized Graphene-Based Materials as Innovative Adsorbents of Organic Pollutants: A Concise Overview. Brazilian Journal of Chemical Engineering. 2019;36(1):1-31. DOI: 10.1590/0104-6632.20190361s20180283

[21] Pérez-Ramírez EF, Luz-Asunción M, Martínez-Hernández AL, Velasco-Santos C. Graphene Materials to Remove Organic Pollutants and Heavy Metals from Water: Photocatalysis and Adsorption. In: Cao W, editor. Semiconductor Photocatalysis - Materials, Mechanisms and Applications. Available from: https://www.intechopen.com/books/semiconductor-photocatalysis-materials-mechanisms-and-applications/graphene-materials-to-remove-organic-pollutants-and-heavy-metals-from-water-photocatalysis-and-adsor: Intechopen; 2016. DOI:10.5772/62777

[22] WHO. GLOBOCAN 2012: Estimated Cancer Incidence, Mortality and Prevalence Worldwide in 2012. Lyon, France: International Agency for Research on Cancer, 2012.

[23] WHO. Cancer prevention and control in the context of an integrated approach Report by the Secretariat of WHO, 2016.

[24] Fiorillo M, Verre AF, Iliut M, Peiris-Pagés M, Ozsvari B, Gandara R, Cappello AR, Sotgia F, Vijayaraghavan A, Lisanti MP. Graphene oxide selectively targets cancer stem cells, across multiple tumor types: implications for non-toxic cancer treatment, via "differentiation-based nano-therapy". Oncotarget. 2015;6(6): 3553-3562. DOI:10.18632/oncotarget.3348

[25] Wang S, Sun H, Ang HM, Tadé MO. Adsorptive remediation of environmental pollutants using novel graphene-based nanomaterials. Chemical Engineering Journal. 2013;226: 336-347. DOI:10.1016/j.cej.2013.04.070

[26] Loh KP, Bao Q, Ang PK, Yang J. The chemistry of graphene. Journal of Materials Chemistry. 2010;20(12): 2277-2289. DOI:10.1039/B920539J

[27] Lee C, Wei X, Kysar JW, Hone J. Measurement of the Elastic Properties and Intrinsic Strength of Monolayer Graphene. Science. 2008;321(5887): 385-388. DOI:10.1126/science.1157996

[28] Balandin AA, Ghosh S, Bao W, Calizo I, Teweldebrhan D, Miao F, Lau CN. Superior Thermal Conductivity of Single-Layer Graphene. Nano Letters.

2008;8(3):902-907. DOI:10.1021/nl0731872

[29] Gao W, Alemany LB, Ci L, Ajayan PM. New insights into the structure and reduction of graphite oxide. Nature Chemistry. 2009;1(5): 403-408. DOI:10.1038/nchem.281

[30] Nair RR, Blake P, Grigorenko AN, Novoselov KS, Booth TJ, Stauber T, Peres NMR, Geim AK. Fine Structure Constant Defines Visual Transparency of Graphene. Science. 2008;320(5881): 1308-1308. DOI:10.1126/science.1156965

[31] Gulzar A, Yang P, He F, Xu J, Yang D, Xu L, Jan MO. Bioapplications of graphene constructed functional nanomaterials. Chemico-Biological Interactions. 2017;262:69-89. DOI:10.1016/j.cbi.2016.11.019

[32] Gómez-Navarro C, Burghard M, Kern K. Elastic Properties of Chemically Derived Single Graphene Sheets. Nano Letters. 2008;8(7):2045-2049. DOI:10.1021/nl801384y

[33] Suk JW, Piner RD, An J, Ruoff RS. Mechanical Properties of Monolayer Graphene Oxide. ACS Nano. 2010;4 (11):6557-6564. DOI:10.1021/nn101781v

[34] Renteria JD, Ramirez S, Malekpour H, Alonso B, Centeno A, Zurutuza A, Cocemasov AI, Nika DL, Balandin AA. Strongly Anisotropic Thermal Conductivity of Free-Standing Reduced Graphene Oxide Films Annealed at High Temperature. Advanced Functional Materials. 2015;25(29):4664-4672. DOI:10.1002/adfm.201501429

[35] Syama S, Mohanan PV. Comprehensive Application of Graphene: Emphasis on Biomedical Concerns. Nano-Micro Letters. 2019;11 (1):6. DOI:10.1007/s40820-019-0237-5

[36] Robinson JT, Tabakman SM, Liang Y, Wang H, Sanchez Casalongue H, Vinh D, Dai H. Ultrasmall Reduced Graphene Oxide with High Near-Infrared Absorbance for Photothermal Therapy. Journal of the American Chemical Society. 2011;133 (17):6825-6831. DOI:10.1021/ja2010175

[37] Soldano C, Mahmood A, Dujardin E. Production, properties and potential of graphene. Carbon. 2010;48(8): 2127-2150. DOI:10.1016/j.carbon.2010.01.058

[38] Zhu Y, Murali S, Cai W, Li X, Suk JW, Potts JR, Ruoff RS. Graphene and Graphene Oxide: Synthesis, Properties, and Applications. Advanced Materials. 2010;22(35):3906-3924. DOI:10.1002/adma.201001068

[39] Zhao C, Pei S, Ma J, Song Z, Xia H, Song X, Qi H, Yang Y. Influence of graphene oxide nanosheets on the cotransport of cu-tetracycline multi-pollutants in saturated porous media. Environ Sci Pollut Res Int. 2020;27(10): 10846-10856. DOI:10.1007/s11356-020-07622-w

[40] Zhao H, Ding R, Zhao X, Li Y, Qu L, Pei H, Yildirimer L, Wu Z, Zhang W. Graphene-based nanomaterials for drug and/or gene delivery, bioimaging, and tissue engineering. Drug Discovery Today. 2017;22(9):1302-1317. DOI:10.1016/j.drudis.2017.04.002

[41] Bagri A, Mattevi C, Acik M, Chabal YJ, Chhowalla M, Shenoy VB. Structural evolution during the reduction of chemically derived graphene oxide. Nature Chemistry. 2010;2(7):581-587. DOI:10.1038/nchem.686

[42] Cohen-Karni T, Qing Q, Li Q, Fang Y, Lieber CM. Graphene and Nanowire Transistors for Cellular Interfaces and Electrical Recording. Nano Letters. 2010;10(3):1098-1102. DOI:10.1021/nl1002608

[43] Cohen-Karni T, Langer R, Kohane DS. The Smartest Materials: The

Future of Nanoelectronics in Medicine. ACS Nano. 2012;6(8):6541-6545. DOI: 10.1021/nn302915s

[44] Nguyen P, Berry V. Graphene Interfaced with Biological Cells: Opportunities and Challenges. The Journal of Physical Chemistry Letters. 2012;3(8):1024-1029. DOI:10.1021/jz300033g

[45] Artiles MS, Rout CS, Fisher TS. Graphene-based hybrid materials and devices for biosensing. Advanced Drug Delivery Reviews. 2011;63(14): 1352-1360. DOI:10.1016/j.addr.2011.07.005

[46] Taherian F, Marcon V, van der Vegt NFA, Leroy F. What Is the Contact Angle of Water on Graphene? Langmuir. 2013;29(5):1457-1465. DOI: 10.1021/la304645w

[47] Kim J, Cote LJ, Kim F, Yuan W, Shull KR, Huang J. Graphene Oxide Sheets at Interfaces. Journal of the American Chemical Society. 2010;132 (23):8180-8186. DOI:10.1021/ja102777p

[48] Park S, An J, Jung I, Piner RD, An SJ, Li X, Velamakanni A, Ruoff RS. Colloidal Suspensions of Highly Reduced Graphene Oxide in a Wide Variety of Organic Solvents. Nano Letters. 2009;9(4):1593-1597. DOI: 10.1021/nl803798y

[49] Hong G, Diao S, Antaris AL, Dai H. Carbon Nanomaterials for Biological Imaging and Nanomedicinal Therapy. Chemical Reviews. 2015;115(19): 10816-10906. DOI:10.1021/acs.chemrev.5b00008

[50] Zhu S, Song Y, Zhao X, Shao J, Zhang J, Yang B. The photoluminescence mechanism in carbon dots (graphene quantum dots, carbon nanodots, and polymer dots): current state and future perspective. Nano Research. 2015;8(2):355-381. DOI: 10.1007/s12274-014-0644-3

[51] Demchenko AP, Dekaliuk MO. Novel fluorescent carbonic nanomaterials for sensing and imaging. Methods and Applications in Fluorescence. 2013;1(4). DOI:10.1088/2050-6120/1/4/042001

[52] Zhang B, Wang Y, Liu J, Zhai G. Recent developments of phototherapy based on graphene family nanomaterials. Current Medicinal Chemistry. 2017;24(3):268-291. DOI: 10.2174/0929867323666161019141817

[53] (SCENIHR) SCoEaNIHR. Position Statement on emerging and newly identified health risks to be drawn to the attention of the European Commission 2014. DOI:10.2875/996348 EW-AS-16-001-EN-N

[54] Smith AT, LaChance AM, Zeng S, Liu B, Sun L. Synthesis, properties, and applications of graphene oxide/reduced graphene oxide and their nanocomposites. Nano Materials Science. 2019;1(1):31-47. DOI:10.1016/j.nanoms.2019.02.004

[55] Wu Y, Wang S, Komvopoulos K. A review of graphene synthesis by indirect and direct deposition methods. Journal of Materials Research. 2020;35(1):76-89. DOI:10.1557/jmr.2019.377

[56] Gonçalves H, Belsley M, Moura C, Stauber T, Schellenberg P. Enhancing visibility of graphene on arbitrary substrates by microdroplet condensation. Applied Physics Letters. 2010;97(23):231905. DOI:10.1063/1.3527081

[57] Kumar R, Kumar VB, Gedanken A. Sonochemical synthesis of carbon dots, mechanism, effect of parameters, and catalytic, energy, biomedical and tissue engineering applications. Ultrason Sonochem. 2020;64:105009. DOI: 10.1016/j.ultsonch.2020.105009

[58] Acar Bozkurt P. Sonochemical green synthesis of Ag/graphene

nanocomposite. Ultrason Sonochem. 2017;35(Pt A):397-404. DOI:10.1016/j.ultsonch.2016.10.018

[59] Gurunathan S, Han JW, Kim JH. Green chemistry approach for the synthesis of biocompatible graphene. Int J Nanomedicine. 2013;8:2719-2732. DOI: 10.2147/IJN.S45174

[60] Gürünlü B, Taşdelen Yücedağ Ç, Bayramoğlu MR. Green Synthesis of Graphene from Graphite in Molten Salt Medium. Journal of Nanomaterials. 2020;2020:7029601. DOI:10.1155/2020/7029601

[61] Pei S, Wei Q, Huang K, Cheng H-M, Ren W. Green synthesis of graphene oxide by seconds timescale water electrolytic oxidation. Nature Communications. 2018;9(1):145. DOI: 10.1038/s41467-017-02479-z

[62] Kar S, Saha S, Dutta S, Rana D, Sadhukhan S, Ghosh TK. A Comprehensive Review over Green Synthesis of Graphene. International Journal of Research and Scientific Innovation (IJRSI). 2018;V(VII):1-12.

[63] Thakur S, Karak N. Green reduction of graphene oxide by aqueous phytoextracts. Carbon. 2012;50(14): 5331-5339. DOI:10.1016/j.carbon.2012.07.023

[64] Wang Y, Shi Z, Yin J. Facile Synthesis of Soluble Graphene via a Green Reduction of Graphene Oxide in Tea Solution and Its Biocomposites. ACS Applied Materials & Interfaces. 2011;3(4):1127-1133. DOI:10.1021/am1012613

[65] Akhavan O, Kalaee M, Alavi ZS, Ghiasi SMA, Esfandiar A. Increasing the antioxidant activity of green tea polyphenols in the presence of iron for the reduction of graphene oxide. Carbon. 2012;50(8):3015-3025. DOI: 10.1016/j.carbon.2012.02.087

[66] Salas EC, Sun Z, Lüttge A, Tour JM. Reduction of Graphene Oxide via Bacterial Respiration. ACS Nano. 2010;4(8):4852-4856. DOI:10.1021/nn101081t

[67] Gao J, Liu F, Liu Y, Ma N, Wang Z, Zhang X. Environment-Friendly Method To Produce Graphene That Employs Vitamin C and Amino Acid. Chemistry of Materials. 2010;22(7): 2213-2218. DOI:10.1021/cm902635j

[68] Esfandiar A, Akhavan O, Irajizad A. Melatonin as a powerful bio-antioxidant for reduction of graphene oxide. Journal of Materials Chemistry. 2011;21(29): 10907-10914. DOI:10.1039/C1JM10151J

[69] Akhavan O, Ghaderi E, Aghayee S, Fereydooni Y, Talebi A. The use of a glucose-reduced graphene oxide suspension for photothermal cancer therapy. Journal of Materials Chemistry. 2012;22(27):13773-13781. DOI:10.1039/C2JM31396K

[70] Iravani S, Varma RS. Green synthesis, biomedical and biotechnological applications of carbon and graphene quantum dots. A review. Environmental Chemistry Letters. 2020; 18(3):703-727. DOI:10.1007/s10311-020-00984-0

[71] Chen W, Shen J, Lv G, Li D, Hu Y, Zhou C, Liu X, Dai Z. Green Synthesis of Graphene Quantum Dots from Cotton Cellulose. ChemistrySelect. 2019;4(10):2898-2902. DOI:10.1002/slct.201803512

[72] de Menezes FD, Dos Reis SRR, Pinto SR, Portilho FL, do Vale Chaves EMF, Helal-Neto E, da Silva de Barros AO, Alencar LMR, de Menezes AS, Dos Santos CC, Saraiva-Souza A, Perini JA, Machado DE, Felzenswalb I, Araujo-Lima CF, Sukhanova A, Nabiev I, Santos-Oliveira R. Graphene quantum dots unraveling: Green synthesis, characterization, radiolabeling with 99mTc, in vivo behavior and mutagenicity. Mater Sci Eng C Mater Biol

Appl. 2019;102:405-414. DOI:10.1016/j.msec.2019.04.058

[73] Basoglu A, Ocak U, Gumrukcuoglu A. Synthesis of Microwave-Assisted Fluorescence Carbon Quantum Dots Using Roasted-Chickpeas and its Applications for Sensitive and Selective Detection of Fe (3+) Ions. J Fluoresc. 2020;30(3): 515-526. DOI:10.1007/s10895-019-02428-7

[74] Chen W, Li D, Tian L, Xiang W, Wang T, Hu W, Hu Y, Chen S, Chen J, Dai Z. Synthesis of graphene quantum dots from natural polymer starch for cell imaging. Green Chemistry. 2018;20(19): 4438-4442. DOI:10.1039/C8GC02106F

[75] Gu J, Hu MJ, Guo QQ, Ding ZF, Sun XL, Yang J. High-yield synthesis of graphene quantum dots with strong green photoluminescence. RSC Advances. 2014;4(91):50141-50144. DOI:10.1039/C4RA10011E

[76] Liu Q, Zhang J, He H, Huang G, Xing B, Jia J, Zhang C. Green Preparation of High Yield Fluorescent Graphene Quantum Dots from Coal-Tar-Pitch by Mild Oxidation. Nanomaterials. 2018;8(10):844. DOI: 10.3390/nano8100844

[77] Halder A, Godoy-Gallardo M, Ashley J, Feng X, Zhou T, Hosta-Rigau L, Sun Y. One-Pot Green Synthesis of Biocompatible Graphene Quantum Dots and Their Cell Uptake Studies. ACS Applied Bio Materials. 2018;1(2): 452-461. DOI:10.1021/acsabm.8b00170

[78] Augustine S, Singh J, Srivastava M, Sharma M, Das A, Malhotra BD. Recent advances in carbon based nanosystems for cancer theranostics. Biomater Sci. 2017;5(5):901-952. DOI:10.1016/j.msec.2017.02.121

[79] Ding H, Zhang F, Zhao C, Lv Y, Ma G, Wei W, Tian Z. Beyond a Carrier: Graphene Quantum Dots as a Probe for Programmatically Monitoring Anti-Cancer Drug Delivery, Release, and Response. ACS Applied Materials and Interfaces. 2017;9(33):27396-27401. DOI:10.1021/acsami.7b08824

[80] Nie L, Huang P, Li W, Yan X, Jin A, Wang Z, Tang Y, Wang S, Zhang X, Niu G, Chen X. Early-stage imaging of nanocarrier-enhanced chemotherapy response in living subjects by scalable photoacoustic microscopy. ACS Nano. 2014;8(12):12141-12150. DOI:10.1021/nn505989e

[81] Chen H, Liu F, Lei Z, Ma L, Wang Z. Fe2O3@Au core@shell nanoparticle-graphene nanocomposites as theranostic agents for bioimaging and chemo-photothermal synergistic therapy. Rsc Advances. 2015;5(103):84980-84987. DOI:10.1039/c5ra17143a

[82] Chang X, Zhang Y, Xu P, Zhang M, Wu H, Yang S. Graphene oxide/MnWO4 nanocomposite for magnetic resonance/photoacoustic dual-model imaging and tumor photothermo-chemotherapy. Carbon. 2018;138: 397-409. DOI:10.1016/j.carbon.2018.07.058

[83] Shi J, Wang B, Chen Z, Liu W, Pan J, Hou L, Zhang Z. A Multi-Functional Tumor Theranostic Nanoplatform for MRI Guided Photothermal-Chemotherapy. Pharm Res. 2016;33(6):1472-1485. DOI: 10.1007/s11095-016-1891-7

[84] Shi J, Wang L, Zhang J, Ma R, Gao J, Liu Y, Zhang C, Zhang Z. A tumor-targeting near-infrared laser-triggered drug delivery system based on GO@Ag nanoparticles for chemo-photothermal therapy and X-ray imaging. Biomaterials. 2014;35(22):5847-5861. DOI:10.1016/j.biomaterials.2014.03.042

[85] Song J, Yang X, Jacobson O, Lin L, Huang P, Niu G, Ma Q, Chen X. Sequential Drug Release and Enhanced Photothermal and Photoacoustic Effect

of Hybrid Reduced Graphene Oxide-Loaded Ultrasmall Gold Nanorod Vesicles for Cancer Therapy. ACS Nano. 2015;9(9):9199-9209. DOI:10.1021/acsnano.5b03804

[86] Zhang C, Lu T, Tao J, Wan G, Zhao H. Co-delivery of paclitaxel and indocyanine green by PEGylated graphene oxide: a potential integrated nanoplatform for tumor theranostics. Rsc Advances. 2016;6(19):15460-15468. DOI:10.1039/c5ra25518j

[87] Oliveira ACN, Fernandes J, Gonçalves A, Gomes AC, Oliveira MECDR. Lipid-based Nanocarriers for siRNA Delivery: Challenges, Strategies and the Lessons Learned from the DODAX: MO Liposomal System. Current drug targets. 2019;20(1):29-50. DOI:10.2174/1389450119666180703145410

[88] Dong H, Dai W, Ju H, Lu H, Wang S, Xu L, Zhou S-F, Zhang Y, Zhang X. Multifunctional Poly(L-lactide)-Polyethylene Glycol-Grafted Graphene Quantum Dots for Intracellular MicroRNA Imaging and Combined Specific-Gene-Targeting Agents Delivery for Improved Therapeutics. Acs Applied Materials & Interfaces. 2015;7(20):11015-11023. DOI:10.1021/acsami.5b02803

[89] Wang X, Sun X, He H, Yang H, Lao J, Song Y, Xia Y, Xu H, Zhang X, Huang F. A two-component active targeting theranostic agent based on graphene quantum dots. Journal of Materials Chemistry B. 2015;3(17):3583-3590. DOI:10.1039/c5tb00211g

[90] Zou L, Wang H, He B, Zeng L, Tan T, Cao H, He X, Zhang Z, Guo S, Li Y. Current Approaches of Photothermal Therapy in Treating Cancer Metastasis with Nanotherapeutics. Theranostics. 2016;6(6):762-772. DOI:10.7150/thno.14988

[91] Zhu H, Cheng P, Chen P, Pu K. Recent progress in the development of near-infrared organic photothermal and photodynamic nanotherapeutics. Biomaterials Science. 2018;6(4):746-765. DOI:10.1039/c7bm01210a

[92] Shim G, Kim D, Kim J, Suh MS, Kim YK, Oh YK. Bacteriomimetic poly-γ-glutamic acid surface coating for hemocompatibility and safety of nanomaterials. Nanotoxicology. 2017;11(6):762-770. DOI:10.1080/17435390.2017.1353155

[93] Hai L, He D, He X, Wang K, Yang X, Liu J, Cheng H, Huang X, Shangguan J. Facile fabrication of a resveratrol loaded phospholipid@reduced graphene oxide nanoassembly for targeted and near-infrared laser-triggered chemo/photothermal synergistic therapy of cancer in vivo. Journal of Materials Chemistry B. 2017;5(29):5783-5792. DOI:10.1039/c7tb01600j

[94] Khatun Z, Nurunnabi M, Nafiujjaman M, Reeck GR, Khan HA, Cho KJ, Lee YK. A hyaluronic acid nanogel for photo-chemo theranostics of lung cancer with simultaneous light-responsive controlled release of doxorubicin. Nanoscale. 2015;7(24):10680-10689. DOI:10.1039/c5nr01075f

[95] Li P, Yan Y, Chen B, Zhang P, Wang S, Zhou J, Fan H, Wang Y, Huang X. Lanthanide-doped upconversion nanoparticles complexed with nano-oxide graphene used for upconversion fluorescence imaging and photothermal therapy. Biomaterials Science. 2018;6(4):877-884. DOI:10.1039/c7bm01113j

[96] Sheng Z, Song L, Zheng J, Hu D, He M, Zheng M, Gao G, Gong P, Zhang P, Ma Y, Cai L. Protein-assisted fabrication of nano-reduced graphene oxide for combined in vivo photoacoustic imaging and photothermal therapy. Biomaterials.

2013;34(21):5236-5243. DOI:10.1016/j.biomaterials.2013.03.090

[97] Chen L, Zhong X, Yi X, Huang M, Ning P, Liu T, Ge C, Chai Z, Liu Z, Yang K. Radionuclide I-131 labeled reduced graphene oxide for nuclear imaging guided combined radio- and photothermal therapy of cancer. Biomaterials. 2015;66:21-28. DOI:10.1016/j.biomaterials.2015.06.043

[98] Lin L-S, Yang X, Niu G, Song J, Yang H-H, Chen X. Dual-enhanced photothermal conversion properties of reduced graphene oxide-coated gold superparticles for light-triggered acoustic and thermal theranostics. Nanoscale. 2016;8(4):2116-2122. DOI:10.1039/c5nr07552a

[99] Li S, Zhou S, Li Y, Li X, Zhu J, Fan L, Yang S. Exceptionally High Payload of the IR780 Iodide on Folic Acid-Functionalized Graphene Quantum Dots for Targeted Photothermal Therapy. ACS Applied Materials and Interfaces. 2017;9(27):22332-22341. DOI:10.1021/acsami.7b07267

[100] Qin H, Zhou T, Yang S, Xing D. Fluorescence quenching nanoprobes dedicated to in vivo photoacoustic imaging and high-efficient tumor therapy in deep-seated tissue. Small. 2015;11(22):2675-2686. DOI:10.1002/smll.201403395

[101] Wang Y, Wang H, Liu D, Song S, Wang X, Zhang H. Graphene oxide covalently grafted upconversion nanoparticles for combined NIR mediated imaging and photothermal/photodynamic cancer therapy. Biomaterials. 2013;34(31):7715-7724. DOI:10.1016/j.biomaterials.2013.06.045

[102] Jin Y, Wang J, Ke H, Wang S, Dai Z. Graphene oxide modified PLA microcapsules containing gold nanoparticles for ultrasonic/CT bimodal imaging guided photothermal tumor therapy. Biomaterials. 2013;34(20):4794-4802. DOI:10.1016/j.biomaterials.2013.03.027

[103] Ma X, Qu Q, Zhao Y, Luo Z, Zhao Y, Ng KW, Zhao Y. Graphene oxide wrapped gold nanoparticles for intracellular Raman imaging and drug delivery. Journal of Materials Chemistry B. 2013;1(47):6495-6500. DOI:10.1039/C3TB21385D

[104] Chen Y-W, Liu T-Y, Chen P-J, Chang P-H, Chen S-Y. A High-Sensitivity and Low-Power Theranostic Nanosystem for Cell SERS Imaging and Selectively Photothermal Therapy Using Anti-EGFR-Conjugated Reduced Graphene Oxide/Mesoporous Silica/AuNPs Nanosheets. Small. 2016;12(11):1458-1468. DOI:10.1002/smll.201502917

[105] Gao S, Zhang L, Wang G, Yang K, Chen M, Tian R, Ma Q, Zhu L. Hybrid graphene/Au activatable theranostic agent for multimodalities imaging guided enhanced photothermal therapy. Biomaterials. 2016;79:36-45. DOI:10.1016/j.biomaterials.2015.11.041

[106] Miao W, Shim G, Kim G, Lee S, Lee HJ, Kim YB, Byun Y, Oh YK. Image-guided synergistic photothermal therapy using photoresponsive imaging agent-loaded graphene-based nanosheets. Journal of controlled release : official journal of the Controlled Release Society. 2015;211:28-36. DOI:10.1016/j.jconrel.2015.05.280

[107] Zheng A, Zhang D, Wu M, Yang H, Liu X, Liu J. Multifunctional human serum albumin-modified reduced graphene oxide for targeted photothermal therapy of hepatocellular carcinoma. Rsc Advances. 2016;6(14):11167-11175. DOI:10.1039/c5ra24785c

[108] Wu C, Li D, Wang L, Guan X, Tian Y, Yang H, Li S, Liu Y. Single wavelength light-mediated, synergistic bimodal cancer photoablation and amplified photothermal performance by graphene/gold nanostar/photosensitizer theranostics. Acta

Biomaterialia. 2017;53:631-642. DOI: 10.1016/j.actbio.2017.01.078

[109] Nergiz SZ, Gandra N, Tadepalli S, Singamaneni S. Multifunctional Hybrid Nanopatches of Graphene Oxide and Gold Nanostars for Ultraefficient Photothermal Cancer Therapy. ACS Applied Materials & Interfaces. 2014;6(18):16395-16402. DOI:10.1021/am504795d

[110] Rong P, Wu J, Liu Z, Ma X, Yu L, Zhou K, Zeng W, Wang W. Fluorescence dye loaded nano-graphene for multimodal imaging guided photothermal therapy. RSC Advances. 2016;6(3):1894-1901. DOI:10.1039/C5RA24752G

[111] Wang Y-W, Fu Y-Y, Peng Q, Guo S-S, Liu G, Li J, Yang H-H, Chen G-N. Dye-enhanced graphene oxide for photothermal therapy and photoacoustic imaging. Journal of Materials Chemistry B. 2013;1(42): 5762-5767. DOI:10.1039/C3TB20986E

[112] Yu J, Lin YH, Yang L, Huang CC, Chen L, Wang WC, Chen GW, Yan J, Sawettanun S, Lin CH. Improved Anticancer Photothermal Therapy Using the Bystander Effect Enhanced by Antiarrhythmic Peptide Conjugated Dopamine-Modified Reduced Graphene Oxide Nanocomposite. Adv Healthc Mater. 2017;6(2). DOI:10.1002/adhm.201600804

[113] Huang G, Zhu X, Li H, Wang L, Chi X, Chen J, Wang X, Chen Z, Gao J. Facile integration of multiple magnetite nanoparticles for theranostics combining efficient MRI and thermal therapy. Nanoscale. 2015;7(6): 2667-2675. DOI:10.1039/c4nr06616b

[114] Tabish TA, Zhang S, Winyard PG. Developing the next generation of graphene-based platforms for cancer therapeutics: The potential role of reactive oxygen species. Redox Biology. 2018;15:34-40. DOI:10.1016/j.redox.2017.11.018

[115] Cao Y, Dong H, Yang Z, Zhong X, Chen Y, Dai W, Zhang X. Aptamer-Conjugated Graphene Quantum Dots/Porphyrin Derivative Theranostic Agent for Intracellular Cancer-Related MicroRNA Detection and Fluorescence-Guided Photothermal/Photodynamic Synergetic Therapy. ACS applied materials & interfaces. 2017;9(1): 159-166. DOI:10.1021/acsami.6b13150

[116] Viraka Nellore BP, Pramanik A, Chavva SR, Sinha SS, Robinson C, Fan Z, Kanchanapally R, Grennell J, Weaver I, Hamme AT, Ray PC. Aptamer-conjugated theranostic hybrid graphene oxide with highly selective biosensing and combined therapy capability. Faraday Discuss. 2014;175: 257-271. DOI:10.1039/c4fd00074a

[117] Battogtokh G, Ko YT. Graphene oxide-incorporated pH-responsive folate-albumin-photosensitizer nanocomplex as image-guided dual therapeutics. Journal of controlled release : official journal of the Controlled Release Society. 2016;234:10-20. DOI: 10.1016/j.jconrel.2016.05.007

[118] Cho Y, Kim H, Choi Y. A graphene oxide-photosensitizer complex as an enzyme-activatable theranostic agent. Chemical communications (Cambridge, England). 2013;49(12):1202-1204. DOI: 10.1039/c2cc36297j

[119] Luo S, Yang Z, Tan X, Wang Y, Zeng Y, Wang Y, Li C, Li R, Shi C. Multifunctional Photosensitizer Grafted on Polyethylene Glycol and Polyethylenimine Dual-Functionalized Nanographene Oxide for Cancer-Targeted Near-Infrared Imaging and Synergistic Phototherapy. ACS Applied Materials and Interfaces. 2016;8(27): 17176-17186. DOI:10.1021/acsami.6b05383

[120] Kalluru P, Vankayala R, Chiang C-S, Hwang KC. Nano-graphene oxide-mediated In vivo fluorescence imaging and bimodal photodynamic and

photothermal destruction of tumors. Biomaterials. 2016;95:1-10. DOI: 10.1016/j.biomaterials.2016.04.006

[121] Gulzar A, Xu J, Yang D, Xu L, He F, Gai S, Yang P. Nano-graphene oxide-UCNP-Ce6 covalently constructed nanocomposites for NIR-mediated bioimaging and PTT/PDT combinatorial therapy. Dalton transactions (Cambridge, England : 2003). 2018;47(11):3931-3939. DOI:10.1039/c7dt04141a

[122] Yan X, Hu H, Lin J, Jin AJ, Niu G, Zhang S, Huang P, Shen B, Chen X. Optical and photoacoustic dual-modality imaging guided synergistic photodynamic/photothermal therapies. Nanoscale. 2015;7(6):2520-2526. DOI: 10.1039/c4nr06868h

[123] Taratula O, Patel M, Schumann C, Naleway MA, Pang AJ, He H, Taratula O. Phthalocyanine-loaded graphene nanoplatform for imaging-guided combinatorial phototherapy. Int J Nanomedicine. 2015;10:2347-2362. DOI:10.2147/ijn.s81097

[124] Bi H, He F, Dai Y, Xu J, Dong Y, Yang D, Gai S, Li L, Li C, Yang P. Quad-Model Imaging-Guided High-Efficiency Phototherapy Based on Upconversion Nanoparticles and ZnFe2O4 Integrated Graphene Oxide. Inorganic Chemistry. 2018;57(16):9988-9998. DOI:10.1021/acs.inorgchem.8b01159

[125] Ko NR, Nafiujjaman M, Lee JS, Lim HN, Lee YK, Kwon IK. Graphene quantum dot-based theranostic agents for active targeting of breast cancer. Rsc Advances. 2017;7(19):11420-11427. DOI: 10.1039/c6ra25949a

[126] Thakur M, Mewada A, Pandey S, Bhori M, Singh K, Sharon M, Sharon M. Milk-derived multi-fluorescent graphene quantum dot-based cancer theranostic system. Materials science & engineering C, Materials for biological applications. 2016;67:468-477. DOI: 10.1016/j.msec.2016.05.007

[127] Zhou L, Zhou L, Ge X, Zhou J, Wei S, Shen J. Multicolor imaging and the anticancer effect of a bifunctional silica nanosystem based on the complex of graphene quantum dots and hypocrellin A. Chemical communications (Cambridge, England). 2015;51(2): 421-424. DOI:10.1039/c4cc06968d

[128] Nurunnabi M, Khatun Z, Reeck GR, Lee DY, Lee Y-k. Photoluminescent Graphene Nanoparticles for Cancer Phototherapy and Imaging. ACS Applied Materials & Interfaces. 2014;6(15):12413-12421. DOI:10.1021/am504071z

[129] Ge J, Lan M, Zhou B, Liu W, Guo L, Wang H, Jia Q, Niu G, Huang X, Zhou H, Meng X, Wang P, Lee C-S, Zhang W, Han X. A graphene quantum dot photodynamic therapy agent with high singlet oxygen generation. Nature Communications. 2014;5(1):4596. DOI: 10.1038/ncomms5596

[130] Su X, Chan C, Shi J, Tsang MK, Pan Y, Cheng C, Gerile O, Yang M. A graphene quantum dot@Fe(3)O(4)@SiO(2) based nanoprobe for drug delivery sensing and dual-modal fluorescence and MRI imaging in cancer cells. Biosens Bioelectron. 2017;92: 489-495. DOI:10.1016/j.bios.2016.10.076

[131] Su Y-L, Yu T-W, Chiang W-H, Chiu H-C, Chang C-H, Chiang C-S, Hu S-H. Hierarchically Targeted and Penetrated Delivery of Drugs to Tumors by Size-Changeable Graphene Quantum Dot Nanoaircrafts for Photolytic Therapy. Advanced Functional Materials. 2017;27(23). DOI:10.1002/adfm.201700056

[132] Zhang Y, Zhang H, Wang Y, Wu H, Zeng B, Zhang Y, Tian Q, Yang S. Hydrophilic graphene oxide/bismuth selenide nanocomposites for CT imaging, photoacoustic imaging, and photothermal therapy. Journal of Materials Chemistry B. 2017;5(9): 1846-1855. DOI:10.1039/c6tb02137a

[133] Song S, He S, Tao Y, Wang L, Han F, Chen H, Zhang Z. Indocyanine Green Loaded Magnetic Carbon Nanoparticles for Near Infrared Fluorescence/Magnetic Resonance Dual-Modal Imaging and Photothermal Therapy of Tumor. ACS Applied Materials & Interfaces. 2017;9 (11):9484-9495. DOI:10.1021/acsami.7b00490

[134] Zhang J, Hu D, Cui H, Gao G, Sheng Z, Cai L. Indocyanine green-loaded polydopamine coated reduced graphene oxide for theranostic applications. Nanomedicine-Nanotechnology Biology and Medicine. 2016;12(2):516-516. DOI: 10.1016/j.nano.2015.12.197

[135] Siddiqui SI, Chaudhry SA. A review on graphene oxide and its composites preparation and their use for the removal of As3+and As5+ from water under the effect of various parameters: Application of isotherm, kinetic and thermodynamics. Process Safety and Environmental Protection. 2018;119: 138-163. DOI:10.1016/j.psep.2018.07.020

[136] Baragano D, Forjan R, Welte L, Gallego JLR. Nanoremediation of As and metals polluted soils by means of graphene oxide nanoparticles. Sci Rep. 2020;10(1):1896. DOI:10.1038/s41598-020-58852-4

[137] Li Y, Zhang P, Du Q, Peng X, Liu T, Wang Z, Xia Y, Zhang W, Wang K, Zhu H, Wu D. Adsorption of fluoride from aqueous solution by graphene. J Colloid Interface Sci. 2011; 363(1):348-354. DOI:10.1016/j.jcis.2011.07.032

[138] Paramasivan T, Sivarajasekar N, Muthusaravanan S, Subashini R, Prakashmaran J, Sivamani S, Ajmal Koya P. Graphene Family Materials for the Removal of Pesticides from Water. A New Generation Material Graphene: Applications in Water Technology2019. p. 309-327. DOI:10.1007/978-3-319-75484-0_13

Chapter 6

Regulation of Angiogenesis Using Nanomaterial Based Formulations: An Emerging Therapeutic Strategy to Manage Multiple Pathological Conditions

Aswini Poyyakkara, Sruthi Thekkeveedu, Sharath S. Shankar and V.B. Sameer Kumar

Abstract

Angiogenesis is an indispensable biological process, any aberrancy associated with which can lead to pathological manifestations. To manage different pathological conditions associated with abnormal angiogenesis, Nanomaterial based formulations have been tested in *in vitro* and *in vivo* models by different groups. The research advancements pertaining to the applications of major candidate nanomaterials for the treatment of pathologies like tumor, cardiovascular diseases, diabetic retinopathy, age related macular degeneration, chronic wounds, impaired osteogenesis and nerve tissue degeneration, have been briefed in this chapter.

Keywords: angiogenesis, nanomaterials, tumor, cardiovascular diseases, diabetic retinopathy, age related macular degeneration, chronic wounds, osteogenesis, nerve tissue degeneration

1. Introduction

Angiogenesis is an important biological process which involves the development of new capillary network from the pre-existing vasculature [1, 2]. The process of angiogenesis is indispensable in supplying oxygen and nutrients to cells under hypoxia, and it has been implicated in different physiological processes such as wound healing, embryogenesis etc. It has also been reported to play key role in many pathologies including diabetic retinopathy and cancer [3]. Angiogenesis is a multi-step process, which commences when the primary, pro angiogenic cytokine, VEGF, is secreted by the cells experiencing hypoxia. Thereafter the interaction of VEGF with its receptor (VEGFR2) on the nearby endothelial cells (EC), leads to EC activation, proliferation, migration, extra cellular matrix (ECM) remodeling, tube formation followed by loop formation leading finally to neo vessel formation and vascular stabilization [4, 5].

The process of angiogenesis is regulated by multiple factors, which may be pro- or anti-angiogenic in nature. The endogenous pro angiogenic factors include growth factors like VEGF, PDGF, FGF, EGF, angiopoietin-1, interleukin-8, placental growth factor, angiogenin etc. The anti- angiogenic factors include endostatin, angiostatin, prolactin, fibronectin, vasostatin, interleukin-12, platelet factor 4 etc. [6, 7]. An equilibrium exists between the pro- and anti-angiogenic factors under physiological conditions, and any disturbance in that equilibrium would result in pathological manifestations [3]. Targeting angiogenesis therefore has drawn huge attention with respect to the therapeutics of pathologies were excessive or insufficient angiogenesis prevails [7]. One of the major approaches in angiogenesis targeted therapy involves targeting VEGF signaling pathway. Humanized monoclonal antibody targeting VEGFA, namely, Bevacizumab, with the approval of US Food and Drug Administration (FDA), has been employed in a combination therapy for the treatment of metastatic colorectal cancer [8]. In addition, an aptamer which inhibits VEGF 165, namely, Pegaptanib has been approved by FDA to treat Age related macular degeneration [9]. In spite of all such interventions, targeting angiogenesis demands much more explorations due to a variety of unresolved issues such as development of resistance to antiangiogenic therapy, lack of adequate treatment for ischaemic disorders etc. [10].

In an urge to overcome the limitations of conventional angiogenic therapy, researchers globally have focused on developing 'nanomedicines' for the treatment and diagnosis of various diseases associated with aberrant angiogenesis [11]. The field of nanomedicine involves the use of nanomaterials for biological and medicinal applications by virtue of their ability to interact with nucleic acids, proteins and membrane receptors effortlessly [10]. In this chapter, we have therefore focused on various research achievements pertaining to candidate nanomaterials that can be developed as potential drugs for angiogenic therapy.

2. Nanomaterials

The class of substances having at least one dimension less than 100 nano meters are called nanoscale materials and the field of science that deals with the synthesis, study of structure, physical and chemical properties and applications of various types of nanoscale materials is referred as Nanotechnology [12]. Nanomaterials usually occur as zero, one, two and three-dimensional structures. Generally, the nanoparticles are comprised of three layers called the surface layer, the shell layer and the core. The core is the central portion of the materials surrounded by the shell and surface layer. The shell layer is chemically different from the core and the outer layer. The surface layer permits surface modification with a variety of moieties like polymers, metal ions, and surfactants [13]. The physical and chemical properties of bulk materials are independent of their size, however, when converted into nano scale materials their optical, physical, mechanical and chemical properties vary according to their size [14]. Such properties include solubility, color, toxicity etc. The major reason for these improved properties of nanomaterials are due to their high surface mass ratio as compared with the bulk [15]. Due to their unique size, shape, structure and solubility they have found application in the biomedical, optical, sensor, electric and energy harvesting fields. Many nanomaterials are already being explored for their use in biomedical imaging [16], bio/chemical sensing [17], targeted gene and drug delivery [18]. We here focus on candidate nanomaterials which are potential nanomedicines in the field of therapeutic angiogenesis.

2.1 Classification of nanomaterials according to chemical composition

Based on the origin, size, morphology and chemical composition, nanomaterials are divided into various categories. In the present chapter we are focusing on some of the important classes that have found applications in biological field.

2.1.1 Metal nanoparticles

Metal nanoparticles are those particles which may be the pure metal or metal compounds like metal oxide, hydroxides, sulphides etc., exhibit size in the sub-micron scale. A variety of metal nanoparticles has been synthesized with varied structural morphology, size and compositions [19]. These metal nanoparticles can be synthesized from various metal precursors and can be functionalized with several groups [20]. The metal nanoparticles permit surface modification with various chemical functional groups and further allow them to be conjugated with polymers, ligands, antibodies etc. The improved surface mass ratio, shape, morphology and functionality, quantum confinement and plasmon excitation make them suitable for the applications in the field of energy, catalysis, electronics, and medicine [21]. However, they show some demerits such as tendency to get agglomerate and chances of formation of impurities due to their high reactivity. Many of the nanomaterials except gold, silver, and platinum exhibits high cyto-toxicity.

2.1.2 Carbon-based nanomaterials

Among the various carbonaceous nanomaterials, the zero-dimensional carbon-based quantum dots (CQDs and GQDs), one-dimensional carbon nanotubes (CNTs) and two-dimensional graphene (GR) are currently the most popular nanocarbon representatives in biological applications [22]. Carbon-based QDs are the recent extension in the nano carbon family with fascinating properties like biocompatibility, resistance to photobleaching and attractive photoluminescence. These outstanding properties make them smart candidates for bioimaging, sensing, drug delivery and cancer therapy [23, 24]. CNTs have a unique 1D nanostructure, with sp^2 hybridized carbon atoms rolled up to design a cylindrical shape. They exist as both single-walled CNTs and multi-walled CNTs depending on the number rolled-up graphene sheets. Due to their exceptional structural, mechanical, and electrical diversities, they deliver remarkable flexibility, strength, and electrical properties suitable for various biological applications like medical diagnostics, sensing and treatment of diseases. Graphene represents the 2D nano allotrope of carbon illustrating a planar graphitic structure with sp^2 hybridized carbon network. Its surpassingly large surface area, easy functionalization and chemical purity makes it a potential candidate for drug delivery. Moreover, it is also widely explored for *in vivo* imaging and cancer detection.

2.1.3 Polymeric nanoparticles

Polymeric nanoparticles are constructed with the aid of natural or synthetic polymers. As compared to other nanoparticles, they offer advantages like non-toxicity and biocompatibility suited for specific biological applications. Although they are used for biosensing and bioimaging, the major purpose of polymeric nanoparticles lies in the field of drug delivery [25]. Biomolecules or drugs are encapsulated into polymeric nanoparticles to obtain a gradual and continuous release of the drugs at the specifically targeted sites.

2.1.4 Ceramic nanoparticles

Nanoscale ceramics, which include various ceramic nanoparticles of zirconia, hydroxyapatite, alumina and titanium oxide have also found potential biological applications. Some of the distinct features like high load capacity, stability and effortless incorporation to hydrophilic and hydrophobic systems enhance their efficiency in the field of biomedicine, however, work on scaling down its cytotoxicity remains to be addressed before its full-fledged use in the biological system [26].

2.1.5 Semiconductor nanoparticles

Semiconductor nanoparticles, particularly QDs have been heavily explored for a wide variety of biological applications like biosensing, molecular imaging, live-cell labelling and drug delivery. They possess unique optical properties like a long fluorescence lifetime and low photobleaching when correlated with conventional organic dyes and fluorescent polymers [27]. Although, the toxicity of the traditional semiconductor QDs is a typical concern that has to be addressed for *in vivo* applications.

2.1.6 Lipid-based nanoparticles

Lipid-based nanoparticles, consisting of liposomes, nanostructured lipid carriers and solid lipid nanoparticles have gained tremendous attention in the field of cancer treatment and drug delivery. These nanoparticles exhibit very low toxicity, can act as a carrier for both hydrophilic and hydrophobic molecules and ensures controlled release of drugs. Due to its versatility and biocompatibility, liposomes are the extensively utilized lipid-based nanoparticles [28].

3. Nanomaterial mediated therapy for pathologies with aberrant angiogenesis

Abnormal or excessive angiogenesis has been reported to be involved in the progression of a wide variety of diseases affecting different organs. For example, aberrant angiogenesis has been implicated to promote diseases like tumor, auto immune disorders and infectious diseases caused by the pathogens inducing angiogenesis and such diseases have been reported to affect multiple organ systems [29]. Further, it has also been reported to be involved in the advancement of skin tissue associated diseases like psoriasis, allergic dermatitis, blistering disease, scar keloids etc. In addition, it has been reported to be the major cause for diabetic retinopathy and choroidal neovascularization associated with wet type AMD, which affect the eyes [29]. Abnormal angiogenesis has also been reported to be involved in the progression of blood vessel associated disorders like atherosclerosis, transplant arteriopathy etc. [30]. The involvement of angiogenesis has also been reported in the progression of primary pulmonary hypertension, asthma and nasal polyps [29]. In addition, it has also been reported in the progression of diseases that affect the reproductive system, which include ovarian hyper stimulation, endometriosis etc. [31]. Aberrant angiogenesis has also been the leading cause for the progression of diseases like osteomyelitis which is characterized by impaired osteogenesis [29]. It has also been reported to promote nerve system associated diseases like diabetic neuropathy and amyotrophic lateral sclerosis, which are characterized by nerve tissue degeneration [32]. The process of angiogenesis has also been reported to promote physiological processes like wound healing and discrepancy associated with that could lead to complications like development of chronic wounds [33]. Different candidate disorders associated with aberrant angiogenesis and the candidate nanomaterials that can be developed as potential drugs for the treatment of such disorders have been detailed below.

3.1 Tumor

The essentiality of angiogenesis in the progression of tumor growth was a breakthrough finding by Judah Folkman way back in 1971, which opened up an era of investigations, concerned with targeting angiogenesis for cancer therapeutics. It has been established that a tumor cannot grow beyond 2 mm in diameter without a steady supply of oxygen and nutrients by means of angiogenesis [34–36]. Therefore, preventing the neovascularisation has been suggested as one of the key strategies for cancer therapeutics. Angiogenesis in a tumor micro environment, unlike that under physiological conditions, is characterized by the formation of immature, leaky blood vessels, resulting in a continual state of inflammation. This happens mainly due to the increased expression of a variety of pro angiogenic factors including VEGF, angiopoietin, integrins etc. and such factors are being targeted for anti-angiogenic therapy. Anti-angiogenic agents targeting VEGF, such as Bevacizumab has been approved by FDA, however, release of other pro angiogenic factors over ruled the efficiency of such mono-therapies [37–40]. Therefore, combination therapies using multiple anti-angiogenic agents were more appreciated to quick fix resistance to angiogenic monotherapy.

Nanoparticles (NPs) could be employed as a vehicle to deliver multiple drugs, targeting different molecules and pathways associated with tumor angiogenesis [37, 41]. The therapeutic drugs are generally loaded on to the NPs either by chemical conjugation or by encapsulation [38]. The NP-based drug delivery can either be passive or active in mode. The presence of leaky blood vessels in the vicinity of tumors facilitates the passive extravasation of NPs with size less than 200 nm into the tumor site by the Enhanced Permeability and Retention effect (EPR) and such NPs are later on cleared by the liver [39, 42]. In addition, limited lymphatic drainage facilitates the retention of NPs at the site of tumors which in turn promotes sustained drug delivery [39]. It has been reported that NP conjugated Doxorubicin [43, 44] and small molecule inhibitors of angiogenesis [45] could accumulate in the tumor micro environment by EPR effect, which lead to the stoppage of tumor angiogenesis and tumor growth [38]. Further, Caplostatin (TNP-470), an angiogenic inhibitor, has been reported to get selectively piled up in the blood vessels associated with tumors by EPR effect which in turn blocked tumor associated vascular hyperpermeability [46, 47]. The Active targeting of tumor vasculature by NPs is achieved by means of ligands presented on NP surfaces. The ligands would selectively bind to receptors which are over expressed on tumor cells as well as on tumor associated ECs, such receptors include VEGFRs, $\alpha v\beta 3$ integrins etc. [38, 48].

NP mediated targeting of different miRNAs have also been tested for their therapeutic efficacy [49]. For instance, treatment with NP containing anti-miR-21 (CTX-SNALP-anti miR-21) has been reported to silence miR-21 in patients with glioblastoma resulting in an increase in the levels of its target gene RhoB both at mRNA and protein levels. Further, NP mediated administration of anti-miR-21 has been reported to inhibit tumor proliferation, induce apoptosis and promote survival rate in the animal model [49]. Exosomes are endogenous lipid-based NPs which are involved in the transfer of biomolecules like RNA and proteins between cells. It has been reported that miR-23a encapsulated exosomes could effectively induce angiogenesis in CAM model as well as in *in ovo* xenograft model by regulating the expression of SIRT1 gene [50].

Different metal NPs like gold and silver NPs have been reported to be effective for anti-angiogenic therapy. It has been reported that gold NPs (AuNPs) are capable of binding to the heparin binding domains of various growth factors like VEGF165 and bFGF leading to the conformational changes associated with the impaired functioning of such growth factors. AuNP mediated inhibition of VEGF was found to be negatively regulating the phosphorylation of VEGFR2. The inhibitory effect of AuNPs on Heparin binding growth factors (HB-GFs) was found to be greatly depended on the size of AuNPs, further, AuNPs with 20 nm in diameter exhibited maximum inhibitory effect. In addition, AuNP with bare surface was found to be essential for the inhibitory effect on HB-GFs. Further, AuNPs have been reported to block of MAPK pathway in tumor cells which lead to the inhibition of epithelial to mesenchymal transition (EMT) and thence, the process of metastasis [51, 52].

AuNP has also been used as the carrier tool for drug delivery. It has been used to deliver an anti-EMT agent, Quercetin (Qu) and AuNP-Qu was found to be more effective when compared to free Qu, in inhibiting cell migration in MDA-MB-23 and MCF-7 cell lines [53]. In addition, recombinant human endostatin (rhES), an anti- angiogenic molecule, which in conjugation with AuNP-PEG (rhES-AuNPs-PEG), when administrated, targeted tumor cells more efficiently and exhibited better performance when compared to rhES. Moreover, the administration of rhES-AuNPs-PEG in combination with 5-flouro uracil (5-FU) facilitated improved localization of 5-FU on to the tumor site with subsequent reduction in tumor size than that in case of mono therapeutic administration of 5FU [54].

Silver NPs (AgNPs) have been reported to inhibit VEGF induced cell proliferation, migration and tube formation in bovine retinal endothelial cells (BRECs). It has also been reported to inhibit vessel formation in matrigel plug assay system. AgNP mediated anti angiogenic effect was found to involve negative regulation of PI3K/Akt pathway [55, 56]. According to a different study, AgNP has been reported to exert anti angiogenic effect by inhibiting HIF-1 in a dose dependant manner [57].

In addition to metal NPs, NPs based on cationic polysaccharides like chitosan has also been explored for biomedical applications taking an advantage of their relatively low toxic nature and high biodegradability and biocompatibility. Chitosan NPs (CNPs) showed anti-cancer effect in the xenograft model of hepatocellular carcinoma by inhibiting the expression of VEGFR2 and thereby negatively regulating the process of tumor angiogenesis [58]. Further, CNPs in conjugation with Ursolic acid (CH-UA-NPs) have been shown to inhibit cell migration and tube formation in human umbilical vein endothelial cells (HUVECs) *in-vitro*. In addition, CH-UA-NPs have also been reported to inhibit the expression of VEGF in hepatoma cell xenografts [59]. CNPs have also been utilized as a vehicle for the co delivery of psiRNA VEGF and pIL-4 in MCF-7 cells which caused relatively huge reduction in the levels of VEGF protein when compared to the cases where the plasmids were used individually [60].

Ruthenium modified selenium NPs (Ru-SeNPs) have also been reported to exhibit anti angiogenic properties, in CAM model as well as in HUVEC cells, mainly by inhibiting the phosphorylation of Akt, FGFR1 and Erk1/2. Further, it has been shown that SeNPs protected with Ru (II)-thiols (Ru-MUA@Se) was endocytosed by the cells by clathrin mediated mechanism [61]. SeNPs have also been used as a carrier tool for siRNA delivery. A pH sensitive, modified SeNP carrying VEGF-siRNA, namely, G2/PAH-Cit/SeNPs@siRNA, has been shown to exhibit high efficiency in terms of cellular uptake, drug release and gene silencing [62].

The cerium oxide NPs (CONPs) have been reported to exhibit anti-oxidant activity and they are characterized by a cerium core and a shield with an oxygen lattice. Chen et al., have shown that CONPs are capable of inhibiting reactive oxygen species (ROS) induced angiogenic signaling pathways [63]. In addition, the nanoceria conjugated with heparin was reported to inhibit the proliferation of human coronary artery endothelial cells (HCAECs) in a better way than that by unconjugated nanoceria [64]. Nanoceria has also been reported to inhibit the proliferation of ovarian cancer cells in xenograft model *in-vivo* [65]. Further, the nanoceria conjugated with folic acid has also been reported to inhibit proliferation and angiogenesis in xenografts of ovarian cancer cells *in vivo* [66]. The anti-angiogenic effect imparted by nanoceria was reported to involve the inhibition of VEGF signaling pathway leading to the decreased phosphorylation of VEGFR2 at Tyr1173 and Y951 [65]. However, a report by Das et al., have suggested that nanoceria might exhibit pro angiogenic effect also [67], making the use of these NPs as anti-angiogenic molecules doubtful under clinical setup.

Silica based NPs have also been reported to exhibit anti angiogenic properties. Silicate NPs (SiO_2 NPs) have been reported to inhibit VEGFR2 phosphorylation and ERK1/2 activation in human micro vascular retinal endothelial cells (HMRECs), thereby inhibiting angiogenesis [68]. Mesoporous silica based nanoparticles (MSNs) have been used as a vehicle for the targeted delivery of chemotherapeutic agent, doxorubicin hydrochloride (MSNs@DOX). MSNs@DOX has been reported to suppress the metastasis of lung cancer cells by inhibiting VEGF induced angiogenesis [69]. Further RGD (Arg-Gly-Asp) modified MSN has been used as a carrier tool for the targeted delivery of anti-angiogenic agent, NAMI-A [70].

Further, MoS_2 nanoflakes containing ZnO NPs were found to inhibit tumor growth in *in-ovo* xenograft model by inducing apoptosis and by negatively regulating the processes of angiogenesis as well as EMT [71]. Similarly, the Tetraiodothyroacetic acid (Tetrac) based NPs have also been reported to be anti-angiogenic in nature in CAM model and in xenograft model of renal cancer cells [72]. Shereema et al., have formulated a green luminescent CQDs, which inhibited angiogenesis in CAM model by negatively regulating the expression levels of pro angiogenic factors including VEGF and FGF. The CQDs showed anti-cancer property *in vitro*, suggesting it to be a potential drug candidate for targeting tumor angiogenesis [73]. The applications of nanomaterials for anti tumor therapy have been represented schematically in **Figure 1**.

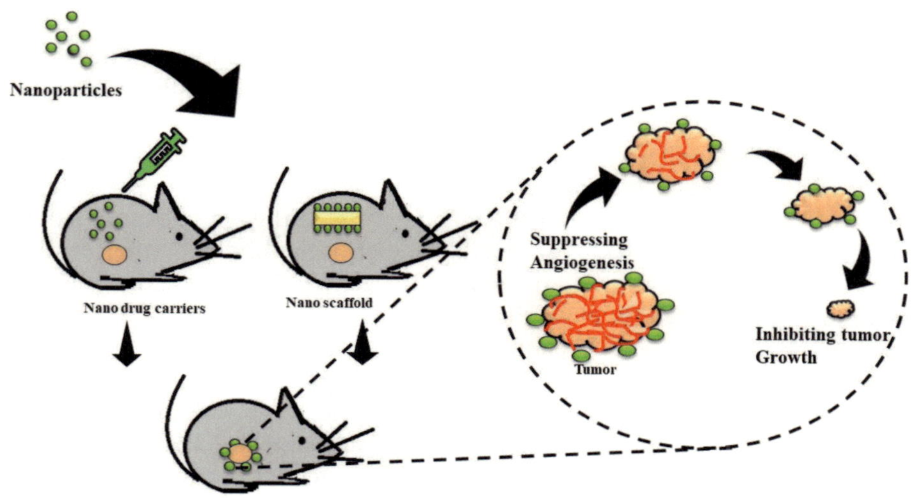

Figure 1.
Applications of nanomaterials in anti-tumor therapy. Many candidate nanomaterials possess intrinsic anti-angiogenic property and few could be used as vehicles for targeted drug delivery. Nanoparticles encapsulated/ conjugated with anti- angiogenic drugs or nanoparticle based anti-angiogenic scaffolds, when administrated in in vivo models, precisely target tumor vasculature and inhibit tumor growth.

3.2 Cardio vascular diseases

Cardio vascular diseases (CVDs), which refer to a class of ailments encompassing coronary artery disease (CHD), peripheral arterial disease, cerebrovascular disease etc., account for the leading cause of death worldwide [74, 75]. Atherosclerosis is the most prevalent pathology behind CVDs, which involves the local accumulation of cholesterol within the walls of medium and large arteries leading to the emergence of atherosclerotic plaque [76, 77]. The process of angiogenesis has been implicated to play key role in plaque growth and intra plaque hemorrhage leading to plaque rapture [78, 79]. The application of nanomaterials has found its way in the diagnosis as well as treatment of CVDs. Integrin αvβ3 has been found to be over expressed in ECs actively involved in angiogenesis, thus, it has been targeted using NPs for CVD diagnosis [80]. For instance, in a murine model of hind limb ischemia, ^{76}Br- labeled multivalent dendrimers conjugated with integrin αvβ3 targeting peptides, were utilized for the detection of angiogenesis by positron emission tomography-computed tomography (PET-CT) [81]. In a different experiment using murine model of hind limb ischemia, a natriuretic peptide receptor C- targeted, ^{64}Cu labeled NP probe was used for the detection of angiogenesis [82]. Further, gadolinium-loaded perfluorocarbon (PFC) NP conjugated with a vitronectin antagonist peptide mimic, has been suggested to be a promising candidate for the detection of atherosclerotic lesions [83]. In addition, PFC NPs incorporated with anti-angiogenic drug, Fumagillin, have been implicated for the treatment of plaque angiogenesis [84].

3.3 Chronic wounds

Wounds are the disruption of the normal physiology of the skin, mucosal surfaces or organs, which occur as a part of a disease or etiology. The process of wound healing is divided into four distinct stages: hemostasis, inflammation, proliferation, and tissue remodeling. Injuries that show delayed healing up to 12 weeks after the initial insult are termed chronic wounds, often it happens because of various reasons such as persistent pathological inflammation [85], complications of ischemia, diabetes mellitus, or chronic venous insufficiency [86]. The application of growth factors has been employed to improve wound healing by promoting angiogenesis, but it possessed some drawbacks like rapid degradation of the candidate growth factors and the lack of controlled and localized delivery system.

Different NPs have been reported to promote wound healing, and many of them were implicated as drug carriers. Studies have shown that different metal ions-based nanomaterials possess the ability to promote angiogenesis and thereby induce wound healing [87, 88]. The metal ions such as Sr^{2+} and Co^{2+} when combined with nano bioactive glass showed pro angiogenic activity [89]. Colloidal AuNPs have been widely studied for biomedical applications due to their unique surface characteristics as well as optical and electronic properties [90]. AuNPs combined with epigallocatechin gallate and α-lipoic acid, reduced oxidative stress and inflammation and augmented angiogenesis, which led to cutaneous wound healing in rodent models [91]. The increased surface area of spherical AuNP helps in electron acceptance and also in scavenging reactive oxygen species that cause oxidative stress and impaired wound healing [92]. Formulation of AuNPs and scrambled peptides were reported to be suitable for angiogenic modulation in *in vivo* and *in vitro* models [93]. Moreover, NPs encapsulated in a microparticle developed by the microfluidic method provided a way to introduce a wide range of proteins including pro angiogenic agents to the injury site [94].

Low expression levels of angiogenic growth factors lead to impaired angiogenesis and wound healing. Heparin mimetic peptide nanofiber scaffolds have been used to overcome this situation, which showed improved vascular development associated with enhanced VEGF production in the treated animals. Also, hierarchically micro-patterned nanofibrous scaffolds with a surface modified nanosized bio-glass have been implicated in improving wound healing [95]. Xie et al. have developed an electrospun fiber nano composites containing different components such as antibacterial polymer chitosan, poly (ethylene oxide), VEGF and PDGF-BB loaded poly (lactic-co-glycolic acid) NPs. They have demonstrated that the application of such a nano composite would prevent bacterial attack in the vicinity of wound. In addition, they have demonstrated that the nano composite facilitated the early delivery of VEGF from the nanofiber and sustained delivery of PDGF-BB from the NPs, thereby accelerating tissue regeneration and remodeling in a full-thickness rat skin wound model [96]. Lino et al. have shown that light-responsive plasmonic gold nanocarrier could be used as a carrier vehicle for the delivery of microRNAs such as miR-302a and miR-155, which regulated the proliferation and survival of ECs thereby promoting wound healing [97].

Carbon nanotubes were functionalized with different side-chain moieties and they were applied for diagnosis as well as drug delivery purposes [98]. It has been shown that the Multi-Walled Carbon Nanotube (MWCNT) supports angiogenesis as the macrophages engulfing MWCNT, produce angiogenic cytokines such as VEGF and MMP9 [99]. Liu et al. have constructed a composite scaffold of VEGF165 loaded functionalized MWCNT, for the prolonged and sustained delivery of VEGF165, and it promoted tissue remodeling and repairing in the *in vivo* models [100].

Graphene based NPs have also been implicated to have massive applications in angiogenesis-based therapeutics [101]. Graphene, graphene oxide (GO) and reduced graphene oxide (rGO) have received great attraction as inorganic additive in biopolymers for developing biomaterial composites [102]. The Gelatin-methacryloyl (GelMA) hydrogel containing rGO has been indicated to promote cell proliferation and migration in *in-vitro* model of wound healing and it has also been implicated to promote angiogenesis in chick embryo model [103]. In addition, ZnO nanoflower based nanomaterials [104] and water-soluble CONPs [105] were also implicated to exhibit wound healing properties by modulating the process of angiogenesis. The candidate nanomaterials which possess the ability to promote wound healing, by promoting angiogenesis have been indicated schematically in **Figure 2**.

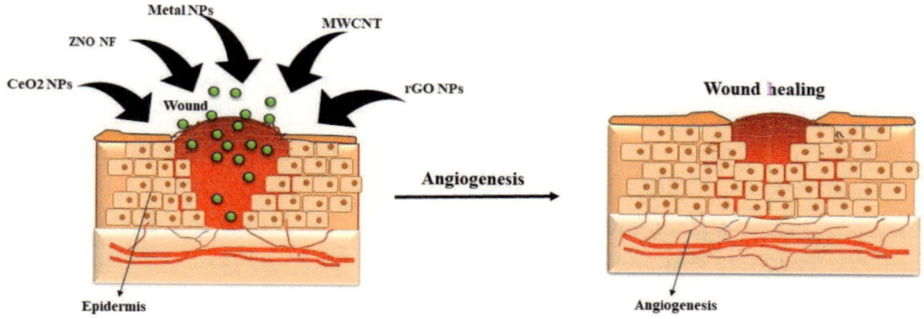

Figure 2.
Pro-angiogenic nanomaterials promote wound healing. Nanomaterials like cerium oxide nanoparticles, zinc oxide nanoflowers, multi walled carbon nanotubes, reduced graphene oxide nanoparticles and metal ion based nanoparticles like strontium ions and cobalt ions, promote wound healing in different in vitro and in vivo models by promoting the process of angiogenesis.

3.4 Diabetic retinopathy and age-related macular degeneration

Diabetic retinopathy (DR) is one of the critical leading causes of blindness and it is a secondary complication associated with Diabetic Mellitus. Diabetes affects the entire neurovascular regions of the retina, with ongoing neurodegeneration, gliosis, neuroinflammation, edema, angiogenesis, and fibrosis [106]. The changes in the vasculature cause perceptible abnormality in vision and lead to blindness. VEGFA, which gets upregulated in response to hypoxia, plays a central role in the initiation of DR. In addition to that, MMP9 has also been implicated to play key role in the onset and severity of DR [107].

The Age-related macular degeneration (AMD) is another complication where pathological angiogenesis is involved. AMD has been classified into two types. The type of AMD which is characterized by yellowish deposits in the macula is known as the Dry AMD, whereas, the AMD with characteristic choroidal neovascularisation (CNV) is termed as the wet type or neovascular AMD [108].

Laser photocoagulation and multiple intra ocular injections are the treatment strategies adopted for the diseases that affect the vascular structure of the posterior eye. It has complications like the destruction of healthy tissues. Though 'introducing protein drugs', was put forth as one of the treatment strategies, it possessed drawbacks like drug instability due to proteases action followed by drug injection. It therefore warranted novel treatment strategies to conquer these drawbacks. So, in an effort to develop alternative therapeutic strategies for ocular diseases, the efficacy of different candidate NPs, exhibiting innate anti angiogenic property or possessing the ability to carry drug, growth factors etc., to specific tissue sites, have been tested by different groups [109, 110].

The AuNPs, as mentioned earlier, possess anti angiogenic properties in addition to their unique electronic, biocompatible, and molecular-recognition properties [111]. It has been reported to induce the nano structural reorganization of VEGFR2 in HUVECs and consequently suppressed angiogenesis [112]. AuNPs have also been reported to suppress VEGF induced cell migration by negatively regulating the phosphorylation of Akt and eNOS in retinal endothelial cells [113]. It has also been reported to obstruct the proliferation of VEGF treated retinal endothelial cells by suppressing Src signaling pathways [114].

Kringle 5 (K5), a proteolytic fragment of plasminogen possessing 80 amino acids, has been shown to be highly effective in the inhibition of EC growth [115]. It has also been reported to inhibit ischemia-stimulated retinal neovascularization in the oxygen-induced retinopathy (OIR) model [116]. But it possessed the drawback of a short life span. An expression plasmid of K5 was encapsulated with PLGA polymer to form nanoparticles (K5-NP) which effectively inhibited VEGF expression and attenuated ischemia-induced retinal vascular leakage and retinal neovascularization in the OIR rat model [117]. Biodegradable NPs loaded with Fenofibrate (Feno-NPs) have been reported to be particularly useful for the targeted delivery and treatment of DR and neovascular AMD. Fenofibrate is a peroxisome proliferator-activated receptor α (PPARα) agonist, which is effective against DR. In diabetic rat models, at 8 weeks after the administration of Feno-NP by one intravitreal injection, the vascular leakage in the retina was found to be reduced. In addition to that the retinal leukostasis was inhibited, and further, the expression of VEGF and ICAM-1 were down regulated [118].

Octreotide (OCT), an analog of somatostatin, is an established neuroprotective and anti-angiogenic agent that targets VEGF. The intra ocular delivery of OCT combined with Magnetic NPs (MNP-OCT) has been suggested to improve the half-life and bio activity of OCT [119]. Polliner et al. have checked the possibility of receptor mediated targeting of NPs to capillary endothelial cells in the retina, and they have demonstrated that Cyclo (RGDfC)-modified QDs specifically bind to the αvβ3 integrin receptors on the ECs and the cellular uptake mediated by receptor binding led to the accumulation of the NPs in the choriocapillaris and intraretinal capillaries [120].

Yandrapu et al. have formulated 'Nanoparticles in Porous Micropaticles (NPinPMP)', by encapsulating bevacizumab coated poly lactic acid NPs into porousifying PLGA microparticles (NPinPMP) using supercritical carbon dioxide (SC CO_2). Bevacizumab is a protein drug used to treat neovascular AMD and it was necessary to inject once in a month intravitreally. The *in vitro* studies revealed that, NPinPMP showed a sustained release of bevacizumab for a period of 4 months. In addition, bevacizumab has been detected for a period of 2 months after intravitreal injection of NPinPMP in rat model, while it was detected only for 2 weeks upon its intravitreal administration in individual form [121].

Likewise, Luo et al. have used, biodegradable PLGA nanoparticles conjugated with integrin-binding linear RGD peptide, as a carrier tool for the delivery of recombinant tFlt23k intraceptor plasmid possessing VEGF binding domains. The nontoxic RGD-functionalized NP delivery system was observed to be getting targeted directly to the choroidal neovascularization lesions after intravenous injection, and exhibited excellent vision restoration in both primate and murine AMD models [122].

Celecoxib is a cyclooxygenase-2 inhibitor, exhibiting anti-inflammatory and anti-angiogenic properties. Celecoxib-loaded poly (ortho ester) NPs were found to be highly effective against AMD and DR [123]. Interleukin-12 (IL-12) has been reported to exhibit anti-angiogenic property by reducing the levels of MMP9 and VEGFA [124]. Zheng and colleagues combined IL-12 with PLGA nanoparticles (IL-12-PNP) and proved it to be exhibiting better efficacy in terms of inhibition of VEGFA and MMP9 expressions in DR mouse retina and rat ECs. Further, the intra ocular administration of IL-12-PNPs showed reduced retinal damage in mice model with DR [125].

3.5 Impaired osteogenesis

Osteogenesis is referred to the process of regeneration of bones, which involves multiple steps such as the activation, migration and differentiation of different cell types [126]. The process of angiogenesis is crucial for the supply of growth factors, hormones, cytokines, chemokines, and metabolites required for osteogenesis. Any aberrancy associated with the vascular supply to the bone tissues would lead to different pathologies such as osteonecrosis [127], osteomyelitis [128], and osteoporosis [129, 130]. Discrepancy in angiogenesis has also been reported as one of the main reasons for the failure of osteogenesis after implantation. VEGF and HIFα are the major angiogenesis related factors that promote osteoblast differentiation and osteogenesis. So, it has been suggested that restoring angiogenesis would promote bone function and defect repair in pathologies with impaired osteogenesis.

Many candidate nanomaterials have been reported to be effective in improving the repair of bone tissues [131]. For example, synthesized chitin–$CaSO_4$–nanofibrin based injectable gel system showed enhanced osteo-regeneration via enhanced angiogenesis [132]. Further, the β $CaSiO_3$/PDLGA composite has been reported to induce the phosphorylation and activation of Akt and eNOS respectively in HUVECs with a resultant increase in the synthesis and release of NO and VEGF. Further the bone regeneration study in the rabbit femur defect model using β $CaSiO_3$/PDLGA composite has shown enhanced angiogenesis and osteogenesis [133]. Nano-hydroxyapatite has been reported to regulate the PI3K/Akt pathway for inhibiting migration and tube formation in HUVECs via inhibiting NO synthesis and eNOS phosphorylation [134]. Similarly, calcium phosphate combined with electro spun poly (lactic acid) has been reported to promote VEGF expression in endothelial cells. It has also been reported to support vascular development and bone regeneration when injected subcutaneously in mice, by promoting the expression of proangiogenic factors like VEGF, IGF-2, GM-CSF, IL-1 beta, IL-6, IL-12p70 etc. [135]. Similarly, Nano bioactive glass, characterized by higher surface area and three-dimensional channel structure, is another material that could promote angiogenesis and bone regeneration [136, 137].

Nanomaterials can also act as carrier tools for different pro angiogenic small molecules and proteins like deferoxamine, adrenomedullin, VEGF etc. For example, Mesoporous silicate nanoparticles (MSNs) incorporated-3D nanofibrous gelatin (GF) scaffold has been employed for the dual-delivery of bone morphogenetic protein-2 (BMP2) and deferoxamine (DFO). DFO, being a hypoxia-mimetic drug, could trigger the stabilization of HIF-1α, and initiate subsequent angiogenesis. Further, it has been shown that DFO could significantly enhance BMP2 induced osteogenic differentiation in mouse and human stem cell models [138].

Ionic components have been utilized for the modification of vascularized bone tissue engineering scaffold. The Copper based nanomaterials could promote the expression level of VEGF, which in turn promoted the proliferation of ECs. Nano-structured surfaces on the Hydroxyapatite scaffolds in copper ion (Cu^{2+}) containing solutions under hydrothermal conditions could affect EC proliferation. Further, the nano-structured surfaces on the Hydroxyapatite scaffolds, promoted angiogenesis and bone regeneration. Dexamethasone (DEX), an osteogenic inducer combined with biphasic calcium phosphate nanoparticle (BCP NPs) scaffold, was found to induce the expression of VEGF and VEGFR2 and supported bone regeneration. The micro-grooves present in the scaffolds managed the assembly of HUVECs into tubular structures and promoted angiogenesis [139]. The gene encapsulated magnetic microspheres have also been used as a promising delivery system. For instance, introduction of VEGF165 with superparamagnetic (nano-Fe_3O_4) chitosan, induced *in vitro* and *in vivo* angiogenesis and bone regeneration [140].

The AuNPs have also been reported to induce angiogenesis during osteogenesis. AuNPs exhibited differences in angiogenic activity based on their surface charges and the presence of functional groups. The Gene profiling data revealed that in comparison with the cells (hMSCs) treated with AuNPs possessing amine or hydroxyl functional groups (AuNPeNH_2 or AuNPeOH), the cells treated with carboxyl group containing AuNPs (AuNPeCOOH) showed augmented expression levels of TGFβ and FGF-2, which in turn promoted cell proliferation over osteogenic differentiation [141].

3.6 Nerve tissue degeneration

Nerve tissue degeneration is a critical clinical challenge that leads to diseases like trauma or permanent paralysis, so research advancement in the field of nerve tissue regeneration is quite necessary. In the recent years, the applications of nanomaterials have received much attention from the research community focusing on nerve tissue repair.

The process of angiogenesis plays key role in supplying nutrients to the nerve tissue which in turn helps to repair segmental nerve defects. Recently, Lopez-Dolado et al. have designed a 3D scaffold containing partially reduced graphene oxide, which when implanted in the injured site in the spinal cord of a rat model, a remarkable induction in angiogenesis and axon regeneration was observed [142].

Further, GO/polycaprolactone (PCL) nano scaffolds have been implicated to promote angiogenesis by modulating Akt-eNOS-VEGF signaling pathway and it facilitated peripheral nerve regeneration *in-vivo* [143].

In addition, Xu et al. have formulated an acellular spinal cord scaffold (ASCS), namely, V-ASCS, for the sustained delivery of VEGF, and it was composed of VEGF165 encapsulated PLGA nanoparticles conjugated with ASCS. When V-ASCS was implanted at the injury site in a rat spinal cord hemisection model, it rendered significant progress in neovascularization [144]. Wen et al. fabricated a hyaluronic acid scaffold with brain-derived neurotrophic factor and VEGF loaded PLGA microspheres, which promoted angiogenesis and nerve fiber regeneration when implanted at the injured site in the spinal cord of rat model [145]. Yu and his co-workers have formulated PLGA microspheres encapsulated with VEGF, angiopoietin-1 and bFGF, and these angiogenic microspheres could release the angiogenic factors in a sustained fashion, which then induced angiogenesis and neurogenesis when administered at the injured site in the spinal cord of rat model [146].

Jian et al. have fabricated a nanohybrid hydrogel containing sulfated glycosaminoglycan-based polyelectrolyte complex nanoparticles (PCN), and it could accelerate neurogenesis and angiogenesis in *in-vivo* ischemic stroke model [147]. Amorphous non-fibrous hydrogel comprised of hyaluronic acid containing high cluster VEGF, when injected directly within the stroke cavity, stimulated the formation of a vascular and neuronal structures, that preceded to behavioral improvement *in vivo* [148].

Delivery of superparamagnetic iron oxide nanoparticle labeled Endothelial progenitor cells (EPCs) was found to induce the formation of vessel-like structures by the production of VEGF and FGF [149]. Similarly, superparamagnetic iron oxide (SPIO)-Au core-shell NPs incorporated with nerve growth factor (NGF) have been implicated to promote neuron growth and differentiation [150].

4. Conclusion

Aberrancy associated with angiogenesis pave the way for the progression of a number of diseases like tumor, cardio vascular diseases, diabetic retinopathy, age related macular degeneration etc. So, targeting angiogenesis presents itself as one of the key therapeutic strategies to tackle such complications. The currently available therapies though beneficial, do possess some limitations like acquisition of drug resistance by cells, fast decay of protein drugs by protease action, off target effects leading to decreased drug efficacy etc. Different candidate nanomaterials were implicated to possess anti- angiogenic properties, which were tested *in vitro* and *in vivo* to explore their additional properties like precise targeting of pathological angiogenesis, cellular uptake, efficacy etc. Nanoparticles have also been utilized as carrier tools for drug delivery. Surface modification of nanoparticles with RGD, VEGF etc. has reinforced them with specific targeting, internalization and sustained drug delivery. Growth factor encapsulated nanoparticle-based scaffolds were fabricated by different groups, to effectuate wound healing, osteogenesis and nerve tissue regeneration in *in vivo* models. On the whole, the application of nanomaterial-based formulations in pro or anti angiogenic therapy is a rewarding strategy for the treatment of complications associated with aberrant angiogenesis, which however, requires more explorations for translating from bench to bedside. The candidate disorders associated with aberrant angiogenesis and various applications of nanomaterials for the treatment of such disorders have been represented schematically in **Figure 3**.

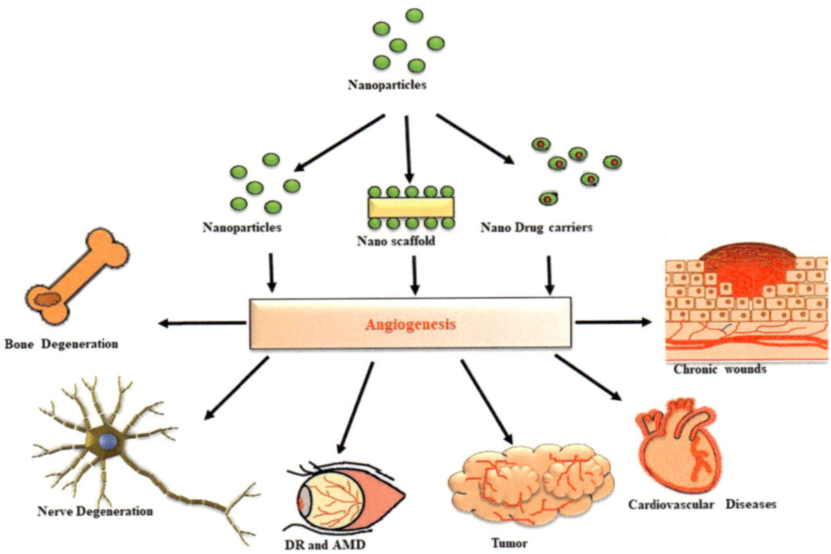

Figure 3.
Nanomaterial based formulations for the treatment of pathological conditions with aberrant angiogenesis. Abnormal angiogenesis promotes the progression of different diseases like tumor, cardiovascular disease, chronic wounds, diabetic retinopathy, wet type age related macular regeneration, bone and nerve tissue degeneration etc. nanomaterials possessing intrinsic pro- or anti- angiogenic property could be utilized individually or as a part of biodegradable polymer based-scaffolds for the treatment of such disorders. Different candidate nanoparticles with surface modifications with peptides like arginine-glycine-aspartate (RGD) and vascular endothelial growth factor (VEGF), could be utilized as carrier tools for targeted drug delivery.

Author details

Aswini Poyyakkara[1†], Sruthi Thekkeveedu[2†], Sharath S. Shankar[1*] and V.B. Sameer Kumar[1*]

1 Department of Biochemistry and Molecular Biology, Central University of Kerala, India

2 Thomas Jefferson University, Philadelphia, USA

*Address all correspondence to: sharathshankar82@gmail.com; sameerkumarvb@gmail.com

† These authors have contributed equally.

References

[1] Ribatti D. The discovery of tumor angiogenesis factors: a historical overview. In: Ribatti. D, editor. Tumor Angiogenesis Assays: Methods and Protocols. New York: Springer New York. 2016; 1464:1-12.

[2] Carmeliet P. Mechanisms of angiogenesis and arteriogenesis. Nat Med. 2000; 6:389-395.

[3] Carmeliet P. Angiogenesis in health and disease. Nat Med. 2003; 9:653-660.

[4] Ellis LM and Fidler IJ. Angiogenesis and metastasis. European Journal of Cancer.1996; 32: 2451-2460

[5] Bussolino F, Mantovani A, Persico G. Molecular mechanisms of blood vessel formation. Trends Biochem Sci.1997; 22:251-256.

[6] Mousa SA, Arias HR, Davis PJ. Role of non-neuronal nicotinic acetylcholine receptors in angiogenesis modulation. In: Mousa SA, Davis PJ, editors. Angiogenesis Modulations in Health and Disease: Practical Applications of Pro- and Anti-angiogenesis Targets. Dordrecht: Springer Netherlands. 2013:55-75.

[7] Gacche RN and Meshram RJ. Angiogenic factors as potential drug target: efficacy and limitations of anti-angiogenic therapy. Biochim Biophys Acta Rev Cancer. 2014; 1846:161-179.

[8] Hurwitz H, Fehrenbacher L, Novotny W, Cartwright T, Hainsworth J, Heim W, Berlin J, Baron A, Griffing S, Holmgren E, Ferrara N, Fyfe G, Rogers B, Ross R, Kabbinavar F. Bevacizumab plus irinotecan, fluorouracil, and leucovorin for metastatic colorectal cancer. N. Engl. J. Med. 2004; 350:2335-2342.

[9] Gragoudas ES, Adamis AP, Cunningham ET, Feinsod M, Guyer DR. Pegaptanib for neovascular age-related macular degeneration. N. Engl. J. Med. 2004; 351: 2805-2816.

[10] Barui AK, Nethi SK, Haque S, Basuthakur P, Patra CR. Recent Development of Metal Nanoparticles for Angiogenesis Study and Their Therapeutic Applications. ACS Appl. Bio Mater. 2019; 2:5492-5511.

[11] Min YZ, Caster JM, Eblan MJ, Wang AZ. Clinical Translation of Nanomedicine. Chem. Rev. 2015; 115:11147-11190.

[12] Jeevanandam J, Barhoum A, Chan YS, Dufresne A, Danquah MK. Review on nanoparticles and nanostructured materials: history, sources, toxicity and regulations. Beilstein J Nanotechnol. 2018; 9: 1050-1074.

[13] El-Toni AM, Habila MA, Labis JP, Alothman ZA, Alhoshan M, Elzatahry AA, Zhang F. Design, synthesis and applications of core–shell, hollow core, and nano rattle multifunctional nanostructures. Nanoscale. 2016;8: 2510-2531.

[14] Mourdikoudis S, Pallares RM, Thanh NTK. Characterization techniques for nanoparticles: comparison and complementarity upon studying nanoparticle properties. Nanoscale. 2018;10: 12871-12934.

[15] Khan I, Saeed K, Khan I. Nanoparticles: Properties, applications and toxicities. Arabian Journal of Chemistry. 2019;12: 908-931.

[16] Nune SK, Gunda P, Thallapally PK, Lin Y-Y, Forrest mL, Berkland CJ. Nanoparticles for biomedical imaging. Expert Opin Drug Deliv. 2009;6: 1175-1194.

[17] Shereema RM, Sankar V, Raghu KG, Rao TP, Shankar SS. One step green

synthesis of carbon quantum dots and its application towards the bioelectroanalytical and biolabeling studies, Electrochimica Acta. 2015; 182: 588-595.

[18] Mohammadi MR, Nojoomi A, Mozafari M, Dubnika A, Inayathullah M, Rajadas J. Nanomaterials engineering for drug delivery: a hybridization approach, J. Mater. Chem. B. 2017;**5**: 3995-4018.

[19] Shereema RM, Nambiar SR, Shankar SS, Rao TP. ceo2–MWCNT nanocomposite based electrochemical sensor for acetaldehyde. Anal. Methods. 2015; 7: 4912-4918.

[20] Neouze M-A and Schubert U. Surface Modification and Functionalization of Metal and Metal Oxide Nanoparticles by Organic Ligands, Monatshefte für Chemie. 2008; 139:183-195.

[21] Ali A, Zafar H, Zia M, Haq I, Phull AR, Ali JS, Hussain A. Synthesis, characterization, applications, and challenges of iron oxide nanoparticles. Nanotechnology, Science and Applications. 2016; 9: 49-67.

[22] Patel KD, Singh RK, Kim HW, Carbon-based nanomaterials as an emerging platform for theranostics. Mater. Horiz. 2019; **6**: 434-469.

[23] Notarianni M, Liu J, Vernon K, Motta N. Synthesis and applications of carbon nanomaterials for energy generation and storage. Beilstein J. Nanotechnol. 2016; 7: 149-196.

[24] Shereema RM, Rao TP, Kumar SVB, Sruthi TV, Vishnu R, Prabhu GRD, Shankar SS. Individual and simultaneous electrochemical determination of metanil yellow and curcumin on carbon quantum dots based glassy carbon electrode. Materials Science & Engineering C. 2018; 93:21-27.

[25] Banik BL, Fattahi P, Brown JL. Polymeric nanoparticles: the future of nanomedicine. Nanomed Nanobiotechnol. 2016, 8:271-299.

[26] Thomas SC, Harshita, Mishra PK, Talegaonkar S. Ceramic nanoparticles: fabrication methods and applications in drug delivery. Curr Pharm Des. 2015; 21: 6165-6188.

[27] Jung D-R, Kim J, Nahm C, Choi H, Nam S, Park B. Review Paper: Semiconductor Nanoparticles with Surface Passivation and Surface Plasmon. Electronic Materials Letters. 2011; 7:185-194.

[28] Feng L and Mumper RJ. A critical review of lipid-based nanoparticles for taxane delivery. Cancer Letters. 2012; 334:157-175.

[29] Carmeliet P. Angiogenesis in health and disease. Nature Medicine. 2003; 9: 653-660.

[30] Van Belle E, Rivard A, Chen D, Silver M, Bunting F, Ferrara N, Symes JF, Bauters C, Isner JM. Hypercholesterolemia Attenuates Angiogenesis but Does Not Preclude Augmentation by Angiogenic Cytokines. Circulation. 1997; 96: 2667-2674.

[31] LeCouter J, Kowalski J, Foster J, Hass P, Zhang Z, Dillard-Telm L, Frantz G, Rangell L, DeGuzman L, Keller GA, Peale F, Gurney A, Hillan KJ, Ferrara N. Identification of an angiogenic mitogen selective for endocrine gland endothelium. Nature. 2001; 412: 877-884.

[32] Oosthuyse B, Moons L, Storkebaum E *et al.* Deletion of the hypoxia-response element in the vascular endothelial growth factor promoter causes motor neuron degeneration. Nat Genet.2001; 28:131-138.

[33] Jenkinson L, Bardhan KD, Atherton J, Kalia N. Helicobacter

pylori prevents proliferative stage of angiogenesis *in vitro*: role of cytokines. Dig.Dis.Sci. 2002; 47: 1857-1862.

[34] Folkman J. Tumor angiogenesis: therapeutic implications. N Engl J Med. 1971; 285:1182-1186.

[35] Folkman J: Incipient angiogenesis 1. J Natl Cancer Inst. 2000; 92:94-95

[36] Naumov GN, Akslen LA, Folkman J: Role of angiogenesis in human tumor dormancy: animal models of the angiogenic switch. Cell Cycle. 2006; 5:1779-1787

[37] Hashemi Goradel N, Ghiyami-Hour F, Jahangiri S, et al. Nanoparticles as new tools for inhibition of cancer angiogenesis. J Cell Physiol. 2018; 233:2902-2910.

[38] Banerjee D, Harfouche R, Sengupta S. Nanotechnology-mediated targeting of tumor angiogenesis. Vasc Cell. 2011; 3: 3.

[39] Peer D, Karp JM, Hong S, Farokhzad OC, Margalit R, Langer R: Nanocarriers as an emerging platform for cancer therapy. Nat Nanotechnol. 2007; 2:751-760.

[40] Ferrara N: VEGF as a therapeutic target in cancer. Oncology. 2005; 69:11-16.

[41] Brigger I, Dubernet C, Couvreur P. Nanoparticles in cancer therapy and diagnosis. Advanced Drug Delivery Reviews. 2002; 54:631-651.

[42] Couvreur P, Vauthier C: Nanotechnology: intelligent design to treat complex disease. Pharm Res. 2006; 23:1417-1450.

[43] Sengupta S, Eavarone D, Capila I, Zhao G, Watson N, Kiziltepe T, Sasisekharan R: Temporal targeting of tumour cells and neovasculature with a nanoscale delivery system. Nature. 2005; 436:568-572.

[44] Chaudhuri P, Harfouche R, Soni S, Hentschel DM, Sengupta S: Shape effect of carbon nanovectors on angiogenesis. ACS Nano. 2010; 4:574-582.

[45] Harfouche R, Basu S, Soni S, Hentschel DM, Mashelkar RA, Sengupta S. Nanoparticle-mediated targeting of phosphatidylinositol-3-kinase signaling inhibits angiogenesis. Angiogenesis. 2009; 12:325-338.

[46] Satchi-Fainaro R, Mamluk R, Wang L, Short SM, Nagy JA, Feng D, Dvorak AM, Dvorak HF, Puder M, Mukhopadhyay D, Folkman J: Inhibition of vessel permeability by TNP-470 and its polymer conjugate, caplostatin. Cancer Cell. 2005; 7:251-261.

[47] Satchi-Fainaro R, Puder M, Davies JW, Tran HT, Sampson DA, Greene AK, Corfas G, Folkman J: Targeting angiogenesis with a conjugate of HPMA copolymer and TNP-470. Nat Med. 2004; 10:255-261.

[48] Xie J, Shen Z, Li KC, Danthi N: Tumor angiogenic endothelial cell targeting by a novel integrin-targeted nanoparticle. Int J Nanomedicine. 2007; 2:479-485.

[49] Costa PM, Cardoso AL, Custodia C, Cunha P, Pereira de Almeida L, Pedroso de Lima MC. MiRNA-21 silencing mediated by tumortargeted nanoparticles combined with sunitinib: A new multimodal gene therapy approach for glioblastoma. Journal of Control Release. 2015; 207:31-39.

[50] Sruthi TV, Edatt L, Raji GR, Kunhiraman H, Shankar SS, Shankar V, Ramachandran V, Poyyakkara A, Kumar SVB. Horizontal transfer of miR-23a from hypoxic tumor cell colonies can induce angiogenesis. J Cell Physiol. 2018; 233:3498-3514.

[51] Arvizo RR, Rana S, Miranda OR, Bhattacharya R, Rotello VM, Mukherjee P. Mechanism

of anti-angiogenic property of gold nanoparticles: Role of nanoparticle size and surface charge. Nanomedicine: Nanotechnology, Biology and Medicine. 2011; 7:580-587.

[52] Arvizo, RR, Saha S, Wang E, Robertson JD, Bhattacharya R, Mukherjee P. Inhibition of tumor growth and metastasis by a self-therapeutic nanoparticle. Proceedings of the National Academy of Sciences. 2013; 110:6700-6705.

[53] Balakrishnan S, Bhat F, Raja Singh P, et al. Gold nanoparticle–conjugated quercetin inhibits epithelial mesenchymal transition, angiogenesis and invasiveness via EGFR/VEGFR-2-mediated pathway in breast cancer. Cell Proliferation. 2016; 49:678-697.

[54] Li W, Zhao X, Du B, et al. Gold nanoparticle-mediated targeted delivery of recombinant human endostatin normalizes tumour vasculature and improves cancer therapy. Scientific Reports. 2016; 6: 30619.

[55] Baharara J, Namvar F, Mousavi M, Ramezani T, Mohamad R. Anti-angiogenesis effect of biogenic silver nanoparticles synthesized using saliva officinalis on chick chorioalantoic membrane (CAM). Molecules. 2014; 19:13498-13508.

[56] Khandia R, Munjal A, Bangrey R, Mehra R, Dhama K, Sharma N. Evaluation of silver nanoparticle mediated reduction of neovascularisation (angiogenesis) in chicken model. Advances in Animal and Veterinary Sciences. 2015; 3:372-376.

[57] Yang T, Yao Q, Cao F, Liu Q, Liu B, Wang X-H. Silver nanoparticles inhibit the function of hypoxia-inducible factor-1 and target genes: Insight into the cytotoxicity and antiangiogenesis. International Journal of Nanomedicine. 2016; 11:6679.

[58] Xu Y, Wen Z, Xu Z. Chitosan nanoparticles inhibit the growth of human hepatocellular carcinoma xenografts through an antiangiogenic mechanism. Anticancer Research. 2009; 29:5103-5109.

[59] Jin H, Pi J, Yang F, et al. Ursolic acid-loaded chitosan nanoparticles induce potent anti-angiogenesis in tumor. Applied Microbiology and Biotechnology. 2016; 100:6643-6652.

[60] Şalva E, Turan SO, Kabasakal L, Alan S, Özkan N, Eren F, Akbuğa J. Investigation of the therapeutic efficacy of codelivery of psiRNA-Vascular endothelial growth factor and pIL-4 into chitosan nanoparticles in the Breast tumor model. Journal of Pharmaceutical Sciences. 2014; 103:785-795.

[61] Sun D, Liu Y, Yu Q, et al. Inhibition of tumor growth and vasculature and fluorescence imaging using functionalized ruthenium-thiol protected selenium nanoparticles. Biomaterials. 2014; 35:1572-1583.

[62] Yu Q, Liu Y, Cao C, Le F, Qin X, Sun D, Liu J. The use of Ph sensitive functional selenium nanoparticles shows enhanced in vivo VEGF-siRNA silencing and fluorescence imaging. Nanoscale. 2014; 6: 9279-9292.

[63] Chen J, Patil S, Seal S, McGinnis JF. Rare earth nanoparticles prevent retinal degeneration induced by intracellular peroxides. Nature Nanotechnology. 2006; 1:142-150.

[64] Lord MS, Tsoi B, Gunawan C, Teoh WY, Amal R, Whitelock JM. Anti-angiogenic activity of heparin functionalised cerium oxide nanoparticles. Biomaterials. 2013; 34:8808-8818.

[65] Giri S, Karakoti A, Graham RP, et al. Nanoceria: A rare-earth nanoparticle as a novel antiangiogenic therapeutic agent

in ovarian cancer. PLoS ONE. 2013; 8: e54578.

[66] Hijaz M, Das S, Mert I, et al. Folic acid tagged nanoceria as a novel therapeutic agent in ovarian cancer. BMC Cancer. 2016; 16:220.

[67] Das S, Singh S, Dowding JM, et al. The induction of angiogenesis by cerium oxide nanoparticles through the modulation of oxygen in intracellular environments. Biomaterials. 2012; 33: 7746-7755.

[68] Jo DH, Kim JH, Yu YS, Lee TG, Kim JH. Antiangiogenic effect of silicate nanoparticle on retinal neovascularization induced by vascular endothelial growth factor. Nanomedicine: Nanotechnology, Biology and Medicine. 2012; 8:784-791.

[69] Zhang M and Jiang L. Doxorubicin hydrochloride-loaded mesoporous silica nanoparticles inhibit non-Small cell lung cancer metastasis by suppressing VEGF-Mediated angiogenesis. Journal of Biomedical Nanotechnology. 2016; 12:1975-1986.

[70] Hu H, You Y, He L, Chen, T. The rational design of NAMI-A loaded mesoporous silica nanoparticles as antiangiogenic nanosystems. Journal of Materials Chemistry B. 2015; 3:6338-6346.

[71] Chako L, Poyyakkara A, Kumar VBS, Aneesh PM. MoS_2-ZnO nano composites as highly functional agents for anti-angiogenic and anti-cancer theranostics. J. Mater. Chem. B. 2018; 6:3048-3057.

[72] Yalcin M, Dyskin E, Lansing L, et al. Tetraiodothyroacetic acid (tetrac) and nanoparticulate tetrac arrest growth of medullary carcinoma of the thyroid. The Journal of Clinical Endocrinology & Metabolism. 2010; 95:1972-1980.

[73] Shereema RM, Sruthi TV, Kumar VBS, Rao TP, Shankar SS. Angiogenic profiling of synthesized Carbon Quantum Dotes. Biochemistry. 2015; 54:6352-6356.

[74] Namara KM, Alzubaidi H, Jackson JK. Cardiovascular disease as a leading cause of death: how are pharmacists getting involved? Integr Pharm Res Pract. 2019; 8: 1-11

[75] Stewart J, Manmathan G, Wilkinson P. Primary prevention of cardiovascular disease: A review of contemporary guidance and literature. JRSM Cardiovasc Dis. 2017; 6: 2048004016687211.

[76] Gallino A, Aboyans V, Diehm C, et al. European Society of Cardiology Working Group on Peripheral Circulation. Non-coronary atherosclerosis. Eur Heart J. 2014; 35:1112-1119.

[77] Ross R. Atherosclerosis–an inflammatory disease.N Engl J Med. 1999; 340:115-126.

[78] Sueishi K, Yonemitsu Y, Nakagawa K, Kaneda Y, Kumamoto M, Nakashima Y. Atherosclerosis and angiogenesis. Its pathophysiological significance in humans as well as in an animal model induced by the gene transfer of vascular endothelial growth factor. Ann. NY Acad. Sci.1997; 811: 322-324.

[79] Moreno PR, Purushothaman KR, Sirol M, Levy AP, Fuster V. Neovascularization in human atherosclerosis. Circulation. 2006; 113: 2245-2252.

[80] Stupack DG, Cheresh DA. Integrins and angiogenesis. Curr. Top. Dev. Biol. 2004; 64: 207-238.

[81] Almutairi A, Rossin R, Shokeen M, et al. Biodegradable dendritic positron-emitting nanoprobes for the noninvasive imaging of angiogenesis. Proc Natl Acad Sci USA. 2009; 106:685-690.

[82] Liu Y, Pressly ED, Abendschein DR, et al. Targeting angiogenesis using a C-type atrial natriuretic factor-conjugated nanoprobe and PET. J Nucl Med. 2011; 52:1956-1963.

[83] Winter PM, Morawski AM, Caruthers SD, Fuhrhop RW, Zhang H, Williams TA, Allen JS, Lacy EK, Robertson JD, Lanza GM, Wickline SA. Molecular imaging of angiogenesis in early-stage atherosclerosis with alpha(v)beta3-integrin-targeted nanoparticles. Circulation. 2003; 108: 2270-2274.

[84] Winter PM, Neubauer AM, Caruthers SD, Harris TD, Robertson JD, Williams TA, Schmieder AH, Hu G, Allen JS, Lacy EK, Zhang H, Wickline SA, Lanza GM. Endothelial alpha(v) beta3 integrin-targeted fumagillin nanoparticles inhibit angiogenesis in atherosclerosis. Arterioscler. Thromb. Vasc. Biol. 2006; 26: 2103-2109.

[85] Singh S, Young A, McNaught CE. The physiology of wound healing. Surgery. 2017; 35:473-477.

[86] Patel S, Srivastava S, Singh MR, Singh D. Mechanistic insight into diabetic wounds: Pathogenesis, molecular targets and treatment strategies to pace wound healing. Biomedicine & Pharmacotherapy. 2019; 112:108615.

[87] Vargas GE, Durand LAH, Cadena V, et al. Effect of nano-sized bioactive glass particles on the angiogenic properties of collagen based composites. J Mater Sci Mater Med. 2013; 24:1261-1269.

[88] Kargozar S, Baino F, Hamzehlou S, Hill RG, Mozafari M. Bioactive glasses: sprouting angiogenesis in tissue engineering. Trends Biotechnol. 2018; 36:430-444.

[89] Kargozar S, Lotfibakhshaiesh N, Ai J, et al. Strontium and cobalt-substituted bioactive glasses seeded with human umbilical cord perivascular cells to promote bone regeneration via enhanced osteogenic and angiogenic activities. Acta Biomater. 2017; 58: 502-514.

[90] Danieland MC and Astruc D. Gold nanoparticles: assembly, supramolecular chemistry, quantum-size-related properties, and applications toward biology, catalysis, and nanotechnology. Chem Rev. 2004; 104: 293-346.

[91] Leu JG, Chen SA, Chen HM, et al. The effects of gold nanoparticles in wound healing with antioxidant epigallocatechin gallate and alpha-lipoic acid. Nanomedicine. 2012; 8:767-775.

[92] Poljsak B, Šuput D, Milisav I. Achieving the balance between ROS and antioxidants: when to use the synthetic antioxidants. Oxid Med Cell Longev. 2013; 2013:956792.

[93] Roma-Rodrigues C, Heuer-Jungemann A, Fernandes AR, Kanaras AG, Baptista PV. Peptide-coated gold nanoparticles for modulation of angiogenesis in vivo. International journal of nanomedicine. 2016; 11:2633-2639.

[94] Zarubova J, Hasani-Sadrabadi MM, Bacakova L, Li S. Nano-in-Micro Dual Delivery Platform for Chronic Wound Healing Applications. Micromachines. 2020; 11:158.

[95] Xu H, Lv F, Zhang Y, Yi Z, Ke Q, Wu C, Liu M, Chang J. Hierarchically micro-patterned nanofibrous scaffolds with a nanosized bio-glass surface for accelerating wound healing. Nanoscale. 2015; 7:18446-18452.

[96] Xie Z, Paras CB, Weng H, Punnakitikashem P, Su LC, Vu K, Tang L, Yang J, Nguyen KT. Dual growth factor releasing multi-functional nanofibers for wound healing. Acta biomaterialia. 2013; 9:9351-9359.

[97] Lino MM, Simões S, Vilaça A, Antunes H, Zonari A, Ferreira L. Modulation of angiogenic activity by light-activatable miRNA-loaded nanocarriers. ACS nano. 2018; 12:5207-5220.

[98] Battigelli A, Menard-Moyon C, Da Ros T, Prato M, Bianco A. Endowing Carbon Nanotubes with Biological and Biomedical Properties by Chemical Modifications. Adv. Drug Delivery Rev. 2013; 65:1899-1920.

[99] Meng J, Li X, Wang C, Guo H, Liu J, Xu H. Carbon nanotubes activate macrophages into a M1/M2 mixed status: recruiting naive macrophages and supporting angiogenesis. ACS applied materials & interfaces. 2015; 7:3180-3188.

[100] Liu Z, Feng X, Wang H, Ma J, Liu W, Cui D, Gu Y, Tang R. Carbon nanotubes as VEGF carriers to improve the early vascularization of porcine small intestinal submucosa in abdominal wall defect repair. International journal of nanomedicine. 2014; 9:1275

[101] Zhao H, Ding R, Zhao X, et al. Graphene-based nanomaterials for drug and/or gene delivery, bioimaging, and tissue engineering. Drug Discov Today. 2017; 22: 1302-1317.

[102] Terzopoulou Z, Kyzas GZ, Bikiaris DN. Recent advances in nanocomposite materials of graphene derivatives with polysaccharides. Materials. 2015; 8:652-683.

[103] Ur Rehman SR, Augustine R, Zahid AA, Ahmed R, Tariq M, Hasan A. Reduced Graphene Oxide Incorporated GelMA Hydrogel Promotes Angiogenesis For Wound Healing Applications. International Journal of Nanomedicine. 2019; 14:9603-9617.

[104] Barui AK, Veeriah V, Mukherjee S, Manna J, Patel AK, Patra S, Pal K, Murali S, Rana RK, Chatterjee S, Patra CR . Zinc oxide nanoflowers make new blood vessels. Nanoscale. 2012; 4:7861-7869.

[105] Chigurupati S, Mughal MR, Okun E, Das S, Kumar A, McCaffery M, Seal S, Mattson MP. Effects of cerium oxide nanoparticles on the growth of keratinocytes, fibroblasts and vascular endothelial cells in cutaneous wound healing. Biomaterials. 2013; 34:2194-2201.

[106] Abcouwer SF. Angiogenic factors and cytokines in diabetic retinopathy. J Clin Cell Immunol. 2013; 1: 1-12.

[107] Penn JS, Madan A, Caldwell RB, Bartoli M, Caldwell RW, Hartnett ME. Vascular endothelial growth factor in eye disease. Progress in retinal and eye research. 2008; 27:331-371.

[108] Salvi SM, Akhtar S, Currie Z. Ageing changes in the eye. Postgraduate Medical Journal. 2006;82:581-587.

[109] Amato R, Catalani E, Dal Monte M, et al. Autophagy-mediated neuroprotection induced by octreotide in an ex vivo model of early diabetic retinopathy. Pharmacol. 2018; 128:167-178.

[110] Bisht R, Mandal A, Jaiswal JK, Rupenthal ID. Nanocarrier mediated retinal drug delivery: overcoming ocular barriers to treat posterior eye diseases. Wiley Interdiscip. Rev. Nanomed. Nanobiotechnol. 2018; 10:10.1002/wnan.1473.

[111] Jahangirian H, Kalantari K, Izadiyan Z, Rafiee-Moghaddam R, Shameli K, Webster TJ. A review of small molecules and drug delivery applications using gold and iron nanoparticles. Int. J. Nanomedicine. 2019; 14:1633-1657.

[112] Cai J and Du B. Gold nanoparticles induce nanostructural reorganization

of VEGFR2 to repress angiogenesis. J. Biomed. Nanotechnol. 2013; 9:1746-1756.

[113] Chan CM, Hsiao CY, Li HJ, Fang JY, Chang DC, Hung CF. The Inhibitory Effects of Gold Nanoparticles on VEGF-A-Induced Cell Migration in Choroid-Retina Endothelial Cells. International Journal of Molecular Sciences. 2020; 21:109.

[114] Kim JH, Kim MH, Jo DH, Yu YS, Lee TG, Kim JH. The inhibition of retinal neovascularization by gold nanoparticles via suppression of VEGFR-2 activation. Biomaterials. 2011; 32:1865-1871.

[115] Cao Y, Chen A, An SS, Ji RW, Davidson D, Llinas M. Kringle 5 of plasminogen is a novel inhibitor of endothelial cell growth. J Biol Chem. 1997; 272:22924-22928.

[116] Zhang D, Kaufman PL, Gao G, Saunders RA, Ma JX: Intravitreal injection of plasminogen kringle 5, an endogenous angiogenic inhibitor, arrests retinal neovascularization in rats. Diabetologia. 2001; 44:757-765.

[117] Park K, Chen Y, Hu Y, Mayo AS, Kompella UB, Longeras R, Ma JX. Nanoparticle-mediated expression of an angiogenic inhibitor ameliorates ischemia-induced retinal neovascularization and diabetes-induced retinal vascular leakage. Diabetes. 2009; 58:1902-1913.

[118] Qiu F, Meng T, Chen Q, Zhou K, Shao Y, Matlock G, Ma X, Wu W, Du Y, Wang X, Deng G. Fenofibrate-loaded biodegradable nanoparticles for the treatment of experimental diabetic retinopathy and neovascular age-related macular degeneration. Molecular pharmaceutics. 2019; 16:1958-1970.

[119] Amato R, Giannaccini M, Dal Monte M, Cammalleri M, Pini A, Raffa V, Lulli M, Casini G. Association of the Somatostatin Analog Octreotide with Magnetic Nanoparticles for Intraocular Delivery: A Possible Approach for the Treatment of Diabetic Retinopathy. Frontiers in Bioengineering and Biotechnology. 2020; 8:144.

[120] Pollinger K, Hennig R, Ohlmann A, Fuchshofer R, Wenzel R, Breunig M, Tessmar J, Tamm ER, Goepferich A. Ligand-functionalized nanoparticles target endothelial cells in retinal capillaries after systemic application. Proceedings of the National Academy of Sciences. 2013; 110:6115-6120.

[121] Yandrapu SK, Upadhyay AK, Petrash JM, Kompella UB. Nanoparticles in porous microparticles prepared by supercritical infusion and pressure quench technology for sustained delivery of bevacizumab. Molecular pharmaceutics. 2013; 10:4676-4686.

[122] Luo L, Zhang X, Hirano Y, Tyagi P, Barabás P, Uehara H, Miya TR, Singh N, Archer B, Qazi Y, Jackman K. Targeted intraceptor nanoparticle therapy reduces angiogenesis and fibrosis in primate and murine macular degeneration. ACS nano. 2013; 7:3264-3275.

[123] Palamoor M and Jablonski MM. Synthesis, characterization and in vitro studies of celecoxib-loaded poly (ortho ester) nanoparticles targeted for intraocular drug delivery. Colloids and Surfaces B: Biointerfaces. 2013; 112: 474-482.

[124] Roupakia E, Markopoulos GS, Kolettas E. IL-12-mediated transcriptional regulation of matrix metalloproteinases. Biosci Rep. 2018; 38:BSR20171420.

[125] Zeng L, Ma W, Shi L, Chen X, Wu R, Zhang Y, Chen H, Chen H. Poly (lactic-co-glycolic acid) nanoparticle-mediated interleukin-12 delivery for the treatment of diabetic retinopathy.

International journal of nanomedicine. 2019; 14: 6357-6369.

[126] Colnot C, Romero DM, Huang S, Helms JA. Mechanisms of action of demineralized bone matrix in the repair of cortical bone defects. Clin Orthop Relat Res.2005; 435: 69-78.

[127] Childs SG. Osteonecrosis: death of bone cells. Orthopaedic Nursing. 2005; 24:295-301.

[128] Lazzarini L, De Lalla F, Mader JT. Long bone osteomyelitis. Current infectious disease reports. 2002; 4:439-445.

[129] Burkhardt R, Kettner G, Bohm W, Schmidmeier M, Schlag R, Frisch B, Mallmann B, Eisenmenger W, Gilg T. Changes in trabecular bone, hematopoiesis and bone marrow vessels in aplastic anemia, primary osteoporosis, and old age: a comparative histomorphometric study. Bone. 1987; 8:157-164.

[130] Alagiakrishnan K, Juby A, Hanley D, Tymchak W, Sclater A. Role of vascular factors in osteoporosis. J Gerontol A Biol Sci Med Sci. 2003; 58:362-366.

[131] Holmes B, Bulusu K, Plesniak M, Zhang LG. A synergistic approach to the design, fabrication and evaluation of 3D printed micro and nano featured scaffolds for vascularized bone tissue repair. Nanotechnology. 2016; 27:064001.

[132] Kumar RA, Sivashanmugam A, Deepthi S, Bumgardner JD, Nair SV, Jayakumar R. Nano-fibrin stabilized CaSO4 crystals incorporated injectable chitin composite hydrogel for enhanced angiogenesis & osteogenesis. Carbohydrate polymers. 2016; 140:144-153.

[133] Wang C, Lin K, Chang J, Sun J. Osteogenesis and angiogenesis induced by porous β-CaSiO3/PDLGA composite scaffold via activation of AMPK/ERK1/2 and PI3K/Akt pathways. Biomaterials. 2013; 34: 64-77.

[134] Shi X, Zhou K, Huang F, Wang C. Interaction of hydroxyapatite nanoparticles with endothelial cells: internalization and inhibition of angiogenesis in vitro through the PI3K/Akt pathway. International journal of nanomedicine. 2017; 12:5781-5795.

[135] Oliveira H, Catros S, Boiziau C, Siadous R, Marti-Munoz J, Bareille R, Rey S, Castano O, Planell J, Amédée J, Engel E. The proangiogenic potential of a novel calcium releasing biomaterial: Impact on cell recruitment. Acta biomaterialia. 2016; 29:435-445.

[136] Kang MS, Lee NH, Singh RK, Mandakhbayar N, Perez RA, Lee JH, Kim HW. Nanocements produced from mesoporous bioactive glass nanoparticles. Biomaterials. 2018; 162:183-199.

[137] Tian T, Xie W, Gao W, Wang G, Zeng L, Miao G, Lei B, Lin Z, Chen X. Micro-nano bioactive glass particles incorporated porous scaffold for promoting osteogenesis and angiogenesis in vitro. Frontiers in chemistry. 2019; 7:186.

[138] Yao Q, Liu Y, Selvaratnam B, Koodali RT, Sun H. Mesoporous silicate nanoparticles/3D nanofibrous scaffold-mediated dual-drug delivery for bone tissue engineering. Journal of Controlled Release. 2018; 279: 69-78.

[139] Chen Y, Chen S, Kawazoe N, Chen G. Promoted angiogenesis and osteogenesis by dexamethasone-loaded calcium phosphatenanoparticles/collagen composite scaffolds with microgroove networks. Scientific reports. 2018; 8:1-12.

[140] Luo C, Yang X, Li M, Huang H, Kang Q, Zhang X, Hui H, Zhang X,

Cen C, Luo Y, Xie L. A novel strategy for in vivo angiogenesis and osteogenesis: magnetic micro-movement in a bone scaffold. Artificial cells, nanomedicine, and biotechnology. 2018; 46:636-645.

[141] Kawazoe N and Chen G. Gold nanoparticles with different charge and moiety induce differential cell response on mesenchymal stem cell osteogenesis. Biomaterials. 2015; 54:226-236.

[142] López-Dolado E, González-Mayorga A, Gutiérrez MC, Serrano MC. Immunomodulatory and angiogenic responses induced by graphene oxide scaffolds in chronic spinal hemisected rats. Biomaterials. 2016; 99:72-81.

[143] Qian Y, Song J, Zhao X, et al. 3D fabrication with integration molding of a graphene oxide/polycaprolactone nanoscaffold for neurite regeneration and angiogenesis. Adv Sci. 2018; 5:1700499.

[144] Xu ZX, Zhang LQ, Wang CS, Chen RS, Li GS, Guo Y, Xu WH. Acellular spinal cord scaffold implantation promotes vascular remodeling with sustained delivery of VEGF in a rat spinal cord hemisection model. Current Neurovascular Research. 2017; 14:274-289.

[145] Wen Y, Yu S, Wu Y, et al. Spinal cord injury repair by implantation of structured hyaluronic acid scaffold with PLGA microspheres in the rat. Cell Tissue Res. 2016; 364:17-28.

[146] Yu S, Yao S, Wen Y, Wang Y, Wang H, Xu Q. Angiogenic microspheres promote neural regeneration and motor function recovery after spinal cord injury in rats. Scientific reports. 2016; 6:1-13.

[147] Jian W-H, Wang H-C, Kuan C-H, Chen M-H, Wu H-C, Sun J-S, Wang T-W. Glycosaminoglycan-based hybrid hydrogel encapsulated with polyelectrolyte complex nanoparticles for endogenous stem cell regulation in central nervous system regeneration. Biomaterials. 2018; 174:17-30.

[148] Nih LR, Gojgini S, Carmichael ST, Segura T. Dual-function injectable angiogenic biomaterial for the repair of brain tissue following stroke. Nature materials. 2018; 17:642-651.

[149] Carenza E, BarcelóV, Morancho A, Levander L, Boada C, Laromaine A, Roig A, Montaner J, Rosell A. In vitro angiogenic performance and in vivo brain targeting of magnetized endothelial progenitor cells for neurorepair therapies. Nanomedicine: Nanotechnology, Biology and Medicine. 2014; 10:225-234.

[150] Yuan M, Wang Y, Qin Y-X. Promoting neuroregeneration by applying dynamic magnetic fields to a novel nanomedicine: Superparamagnetic iron oxide (SPIO)-gold nanoparticles bounded with nerve growth factor (NGF). Nanomedicine. 2018; 14:1337-1347.